This Is a Book for Parents of Gay Kids

A Question & Answer Guide to Everyday Life

Dannielle Owens-Reid & Kristin Russo

Foreword by Linda Stone Fish, M.S.W., Ph.D.

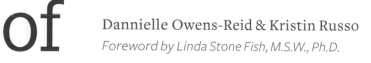

CHRONICLE BOOKS

SAN FRANCISCO

Copyright © 2014 by Everyone Is Gay, LLC.

Library of Congress Cataloging-in-Publication Data:
Owens-Reid, Dannielle.
   This is a book for parents of gay kids : a question & answer guide to everyday life / Dannielle Owens-Reid and Kristin Russo, Linda Stone Fish.
     pages cm
   Includes index.
   ISBN 978-1-4521-2753-8 (pbk.)
   1. Parents of gays. 2. Gay youth 3. Lesbian youth. 4. Coming out (Sexual orientation) 5. Parent and child. I. Russo, Kristin. II. Stone Fish, Linda. III. Title.

HQ76.25.O987 2014b
306.76'60835—dc23

2013040465

Manufactured in China

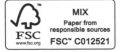

Designed by Jennifer Tolo Pierce

10 9 8 7 6 5 4

Chronicle Books LLC
680 Second Street
San Francisco, California 94107
www.chroniclebooks.com

Dedicated to Sophia and her mom, Carol

CONTENTS

Chapter 3: Telling Others 65

Chapter 4: Thinking About the Future 90

Chapter 5: The Birds and the Bees 115

Chapter 6: Religious Beliefs 138

Chapter 7: Questioning Gender 159

Chapter 8: Being Supportive 187

Foreword

by Linda Stone Fish, M.S.W., Ph.D.

In the early 1980s, while pursuing my doctorate in marriage and family therapy, I became pregnant with my first child; I was both fortunate and challenged. World-renowned family scholars offered well-meaning advice, which, unfortunately, failed to help me conceptualize the landscape of parenting. One professor predicted, "Your heart will sing with joy 50 percent of the time and be burdened by pain the other 50 percent." I wish, instead, he offered, "Let your children teach you who they are as they invite you to join in the discovery of their becoming."

As an academic family therapist, I think about how to best help parents create families that successfully navigate the innumerable crises, traumas, and hurdles of living. Since writing the book *Nurturing Queer Youth: Family Therapy Transformed*, I have traveled around the country meeting with professionals and families negotiating the coming-out process. Countless parents have asked me, "Is there something I can read?" Since my two favorite parenting books, *The Evolving Self* (Kegan, 1982) and *Far from the Tree* (Solomon, 2012), read more like dissertations than self-help books, I have always shook my head, sadly, no. Now I can respond positively, and enthusiastically recommend *This Is a Book for Parents of Gay Kids*.

Researchers and clinicians know that the process of coming out to a parent is one of the most significant events in the formation of gay identity. When children challenge their parents' most fundamental perceptions of them, it can often be a confusing time for the family. The authors of this book guide parents through what can be an emotionally challenging, life-altering event in a constructive way that enhances the development of both children and parents.

This is an advice book with both heart and wisdom. It is a comprehensive, honest, and heartfelt encyclopedia about the process of discovery. Using the experiences of many different families as illustrations, the authors remind the reader that initial reactions will be followed by different, evolving responses. They encourage parents to create a soft landing for children to return home, and they include useful summaries at the end of each chapter to capture important lessons.

Actually, I will recommend this book as a useful primer for all parents navigating adolescence and young adulthood. Spoiler alert: At the end, Owens-Reid and Russo share three essential ingredients to good parenting—dialogue, patience, and reflection. With this book, the authors have managed to give helpful advice that illuminates the unfolding landscape of parenting and helps families successfully negotiate the coming-out process.

Introduction

In 2010, we were nothing more than acquaintances who shared a few common friends. Dannielle, who was about to make a permanent move from Chicago to New York City, had just started the comic website "Lesbians Who Look Like Justin Bieber." She happened to mention to Kristin that, amid the positive feedback, some people were saying that she was stereotyping lesbians and turning the community into a joke. Dannielle felt the comments were off base, and Kristin agreed. At the time, Kristin was on her way to getting her master's in gender studies, so she was more than ready to discuss these issues. Together we decided to start a website where we could address that negative feedback and answer questions from the community while still doing what we loved most: making people laugh. We named the site *Everyone Is Gay*. At the time, we had no idea that we were taking the first few steps into running an organization aimed at helping lesbian, gay, bisexual, transgender, and queer/questioning (LGBTQ) youth.

As it turned out, LGBTQ youth across the world were itching for a place to ask questions. They had so much on their minds and so many things they wanted to talk about, but there simply hadn't been a place for them to express themselves. Our site also accepted questions anonymously, which opened up a safe space for youth to ask questions without having to worry about what others might think. Many kids felt they couldn't open up to their guidance counselors, parents, siblings, or friends without consequences, judgments, or weird looks. EveryoneIsGay.com provided that space, presenting practical and supportive advice to people when they needed it most.

Soon, we began to receive questions, thoughts, and comments, not only from kids, but also from their parents, teachers, community members, aunts, boyfriends, and others. We began to post an answer to a question every day of the week, and after a few months we also added a video element, in which we responded to questions that readers called in. As the site expanded, we realized that there were countless individuals who desperately needed an inviting, judgment-free resource to answer questions and share stories.

Now, millions have explored our site, and we've received more than fifty thousand questions, ranging from the utterly practical to the deeply emotional. We've provided advice on topics ranging from what to do when you've fallen in love with your best friend to how to come out to religious family members. Soon after starting the website, we decided to take our message on the road, and began to travel to middle schools, high schools, and college campuses, promoting equality while still keeping everyone laughing. That shift was monumental, as we were finally able to speak to the many people who had previously been anonymous faces on the Internet. Kids repeatedly told us that we'd helped facilitate a first, second, or third conversation between themselves and their parents. They would watch our weekly advice videos with their families so they could have an easier time talking about things that they previously hadn't been able to discuss; the presence of Everyone Is Gay had given them the courage they needed to be who they were, and to share that with their families.

Connecting directly with LGBTQ youth around the world has given us unique insight into the issues facing kids today. Both of us have our own stories of coming out to family members—shared in the following pages—but it is our years of experience speaking to today's youth that enabled us to write this book. We have seen thousands of youth struggling with how to talk to their parents about their sexuality, and on the other side of that divide, we know there are thousands of parents who have no idea what that process feels like. While we are not yet parents ourselves, we have talked with many (including our own) and have come to appreciate that the coming-out experience can be just as tough on parents as it is on their kids. You may not have expected this, it may conflict with your personal beliefs, you may have concerns for your kid's future life, or you may just need some guidance on how to move forward in an informed, positive way. We also know that, especially in the first stages of the coming-out process, your child may not want or be able to answer the many questions that you have. We are here to help bridge that divide.

This book will address many of your concerns, from the initial coming-out process to how to reconcile your child's sexuality with your religious beliefs to how to handle sleepovers. You'll also hear from parents and children who have been through the process and can share their experiences—both what has worked and what hasn't. As the book is laid out in a question-and-answer format, it will be very easy to find the items that feel relevant to you at any given time. There is no need to read this book cover to cover (though, go right ahead if you feel like it!), and it can be revisited as your experience with your child unfolds. Today you are seeking answers to questions that are very different from the questions you may have a year from now. That is all part of the process. We have also included key takeaways ("The Bottom Line") at the end of each chapter, so there are many ways to digest this information, depending on your personal experience and interests.

While our advice is based on our discussions with countless parents and their children, we, of course, cannot represent the experience of every single family. You may find that our advice helps you enormously in some situations, but that in others, it doesn't work perfectly—and that is totally okay! This book is meant to tackle some of the initial, tough questions that you may have, and to help you begin (and continue) a dialogue with your child, family members, and other loved ones. We encourage you to use this book as a stepping stone toward an even deeper exploration of this process with your child. There is an extensive Resources section at the end of this book to help you continue that work.

There are so many parents who truly want to be able to understand, help, and support their child in any way possible. By picking up this book, it's clear that you are one of those parents. We hope this book can help you feel more comfortable starting that conversation and building a strong, open relationship. This book was written to help you foster communication with your child about their sexuality, to provide answers to the many questions that arise moments (or years) after your child has come out to you, and to give insight into what is often happening on the other side of that divide, inside your child's experience. To help you understand our personal perspectives, here is a look at what it was like for each of us to come out to our parents.

Mashed potatoes, overcooked stuffing, and an antibiotic-infused Butterball turkey: these are the markers of the American holiday known as Thanksgiving. Unless, of course, you were at my house on November 26, 1998. If that were the case, you would have also found a slightly tipsy, wine-drinking mom; a smiling, story-telling dad; a sullen, pre-pubescent little sister; and me at the age of seventeen, clad in Salvation Army–sourced clothing, about to tell my parents that I was gay.

First, some background. Until my senior year in high school, I identified as a straight girl with very close girlfriends and a deep adoration for Liv Tyler. My very observant mother, however, had asked me countless times if I was a lesbian. My answer was always the same: "No, Mom, calm down and stop asking me!" Then, in the fall of 1997, I met a girl. We became friends. We hung out. We kissed. We liked kissing. We did some other stuff. This happened a few times, and then that thing happened. That oh-dear-God-my-stomach-is-squeezed-and-my-heart-is-in-my-throat thing. I liked this girl.

In addition to my oh my God-I'm-gay panic, I was horrified that my mother had been right all along. As we all know, telling your parents that they are right about anything is almost impossible between the ages of eleven and twenty-four. I didn't breathe a word of my gayness to anyone but my close friends for almost a year, which brings us back to the Thanksgiving Day surprise.

Once my sister had left the table, I began to complain about an awful translation of the Bible that had been given to me by a relative. I said something like, "They make it sound like God hates gay people, but that is a load of BS." My mom looked up from her stuffing, her eyes troubled by my angry tone, and asked, for the hundredth time, "Kristin, is there something you want to tell us?" Then . . . it just happened. I dug my fingers into my palm, mustered up as much teenage courage as I could, and answered, "Yes. I want to tell you both that I'm gay."

Silence.

The first thing my parents said to me, and the thing I will always remember, was that I was their daughter and they would always love me. For that, I was (and still am) very thankful. After this initial reaction, however, my mother began what would be a very long journey in reconciling her love for her child with her deeply instilled religious beliefs. The first few years were very hard. My mother and I fought a lot. She cried a lot, and I yelled even more. Through all of it, though, we never stopped loving each other.

Over time, the yelling calmed into a dialogue. She allowed herself to meet my girlfriend. Our conversations progressed, and she began to ask me questions. Slowly, girlfriends were invited over for dinner, and my mother and I found common ground amid differing beliefs.

The thing about coming out is that it isn't one moment at a Thanksgiving dinner table. It is a process that takes patience, understanding, and compassion. It is different for everyone. All we can do is share as much of ourselves as we feel comfortable with and work diligently at accepting who we are, with or without the understanding of those around us.

→ DANNIELLE'S COMING-OUT STORY

I told my mom I was gay while we were making jewelry in the living room. I was nineteen, we were sitting on the floor placing weird green rocks on some sort of thick fishing line, and I said, "Mom, I have to tell you something: I'm dating someone . . . and it's a girl." She immediately screamed, "That's okay, Ellen is gay and I love Ellen!" Referring, of course, to Ellen DeGeneres. I didn't have much of a response after that. She asked me a few questions about the girl I was dating and suggested we make her a necklace.

I think many people have that general sense of relief right after they come out to their parents. For one second, I felt that it was totally over and I would never have to do it again. Oh man, was I wrong. Not even two days passed before my mother called me in tears, begging that I not cut my hair or start wearing tracksuits. While other people might have been offended by her ignorance, I was just scared. I tried to explain to her that I wasn't planning to change anything about myself or the way I lived. It was hard, though, because I was only nineteen years old, and I had no clue who I was or who I was going to be in the years to come.

It took a number of years before my mother stopped asking me to wear dresses and stopped wondering if I was going to end up with a man. She asked me why I didn't want to get married, which confused me because I *did* want marriage; I just didn't want to marry a man (which to her, I think, meant I wasn't really getting married). She wanted to know why I didn't want kids (again, I did). She wanted to know why I didn't want a "normal life." All of her questions really confused me—I felt terrible, lost, and hurt. I thought, "She's right. What is wrong with me that I don't want to be normal and happy? Why am I making this harder for myself?"

This experience was in part why I wanted to write this book. I wondered how things might have been different if my mother had known the effect her words would have on me. Did she know how it felt to be asked, "Why don't you ever want a family?" Maybe a book like this would have helped our conversations, if even just a little bit. Maybe we'd be closer now.

Eventually, with the help of my friends and the rest of my family, I realized my mom's opinions were her own, that they weren't a reflection of my reality, and that I could be happy with who I was—and who I am. I had to go on my own journey to discover who I was and who I wanted to be for the rest of my life, but I know it would have been a quicker and easier path had my mom had the tools to talk to me.

A Note on Our Use of the Word Gay

Identities are complex, and the words we use to describe them are exceptionally tricky.

There are about eight bajillion (rough estimate) different ways in which we understand ourselves, our identities, and our sexualities. Insofar as sexuality is concerned, there are individuals who identify as gay, lesbian, bisexual, pansexual, asexual, and that list goes on. Where gender is concerned, there are people who identify as transgender, genderqueer, gender nonconforming, and the list goes on. (Many of these words are defined in the Glossary, page 215). When writing a book for parents whose children have come out to them as one of these many identity permutations, we had to make a few very difficult decisions. At the outset, we asked ourselves: Should we attempt (and inevitably fail) to include all of these identity categories within and throughout the text? We knew that the sometimes overlapping, sometimes markedly different, experiences of kids questioning sexuality and those questioning gender identity would make it impossible to include answers pertinent to *all* identities in *all* of our answers. While certain concerns (such as, "Will my child always be viewed differently?") address a large range of experience, other concerns ("I feel that marriage should be reserved for a man and a woman") were much more specific.

Given that, we decided to narrow our primary focus to sexuality. Take note: This book, first, is a book for parents whose children are questioning their sexuality, or have come out to them as gay, lesbian, bisexual, pansexual, or any of the other myriad words that represent a sexual identity. However, take note again: Having spent many years in the company of LGBTQ youth (both currently and when we *were* youth), we are very aware of the complexities and intricacies of sexuality and gender identity. Our chapter on gender scratches the surface of what it means to question one's gender, and what it means to be the parent of a child who is in the midst of that questioning. We encourage all parents to read chapter 7, regardless of how your child identifies. We all have relationships with gender, and these are highly relevant and important concerns, even if they don't impact your child directly. If your child *is* questioning their gender, this chapter should give you the first few bits of information needed to better understand what that means, and we encourage you to seek out further resources that focus more specifically on this experience. We also recommend that you read past the gender chapter, as many of the questions and answers contained in the following pages address experiences beyond sexuality.

After deciding to focus the core of this book on sexuality, we were still left with a battle of words. Identity categories, and the words used to describe them, are very specific to the person who chooses to use them. What one person means when using the word *lesbian* to refer to themselves can be very different from what another person means. Some people, especially in younger generations, have come to use the word *queer* as an umbrella term encompassing any divergence from a heterosexual or *cisgender* (self-identifying with the gender assigned at birth) identity. However, many individuals, especially in older generations, view the word *queer* as insulting or derogatory. Words, as previously discussed, are exceptionally tricky. We have chosen to use the word *gay* throughout the majority of this book as a one-word representation of the many, many different sexual identities that your child (or, anyone, for that matter) may use to describe themselves.

CHAPTER 1: Coming Out

Kids come out to their parents in various ways: across a dinner table, in a letter, by text message, or through a song composed on their ukulele. Some coming-out moments happen accidentally; others are planned and thought out for months or even years. Some begin in tears and end in laughter (or more tears); others are welcomed with a knowing nod and a bear hug. Families differ vastly, so there isn't one single experience that you can expect when your child comes out. The one thing all coming-out moments share, however, is that they are not confined to a single moment. Sure, there is the first utterance of the phrase, "I'm gay, Mom," or the first time you accidentally overhear your son telling his boyfriend that he has really cute dimples, but coming out is a much larger process for you and your child, and it merely begins with that initial experience.

The knowledge that this is an ongoing process should relieve some of the pressure you may be feeling as a parent to do everything perfectly in those first moments. If your child has come out to you, or if you suspect that they may in the next few months or years, remember that you aren't expected to know everything. The coming-out process can and should be an incredible learning experience for both you and your child. Have patience when things don't go exactly as you'd imagined—this is uncharted territory!

———

Q: **My child just came out to me, and now I don't know how to talk to them. Help!**

A few days after I came out to my dad he commented, "Hey, so, that Gwen Stefani is pretty cute, right?" My immediate response was to turn the color of a beet, melt into a puddle, and slither underneath the carpet so that I might never have to see or speak to anyone again. Talking to my dad about cute girls was certainly not something I felt ready for at that stage of the game, and the moment was awkward. However, once a little time passed and I became more comfortable in my skin, the exchange began to take on a different meaning. I realized that my dad had simply been trying to connect with me, and I also found it hilarious that he chose pop-star commentary as a pathway to "father/daughter bonding." I now joke with my dad about that moment any chance I get, and I have told the story to countless individuals who are panic-stricken at the thought of coming out to their parents.

—Kristin

A: First things first: it is totally okay that you are feeling confused. This is not only a journey for your child, it is also a journey for you. You may suddenly be faced with many questions that had not occurred to you until this very moment. What will it be like to have a gay child? Will they be happy? What will *your* parents think? Does this mean you won't have grandchildren? Many of these initial questions are addressed in more detail in chapters 2, 3, and 4. As with any other kind of growth or change, though, awkward and uncomfortable moments are going to happen despite your preparedness. Parenting any teenager comes with many new issues that are often difficult to navigate with complete ease, and sexuality, dating, and identity are just a few areas where conversations can feel a bit rickety on their first few go-rounds. These conversations may seem more intimidating now that you know your child is gay, but the key is trusting that those awkward moments are completely normal. Perhaps you accidentally referred to your daughter's new girlfriend as her "special friend," or winked at your son and mouthed, "He's cute," not realizing you were talking about his science teacher. Just like Kristin's "Gwen Stefani Incident," these moments can make for comical stories that last a lifetime.

Now, not every awkward moment is going to turn into a family touchstone, but the point here is that you shouldn't be afraid to say the wrong thing at the wrong time. You have never been a parent to a gay kid before, so this is all brand new. But you had also never parented a three-month-old, dealt with your child's first day of kindergarten, or handled questions about a first dance before those moments were upon you. Parenting is full of first times and involves occasional slips and falls. Parenting is also about growing along with those changes and learning from each experience. If you cause some embarrassment or anger, or you're laughed at for confusing the name of a gay pop star with your daughter's roommate from sleepaway camp, remember that you haven't done anything wrong. You and your child are both navigating an ongoing, evolving relationship.

Overcoming the fear of those awkward moments is key in allowing you to dialogue with your child, and the next step is actually taking the plunge and talking to your child in this new, unexplored context. If your relationship before they came out was one in which you commented on possible crushes they might have or poked fun at them for wearing a polka-dotted bow tie to the dentist's office, try to keep it consistent! If you now know that your son likes other boys, and it fits the way you spoke to him before, you can absolutely say, "So, is John just a friend or is he a *friennnnnnd?*" and then elbow him in the ribs. Sure, he might be embarrassed, but what you are communicating in that moment is that you love him no matter what, and that he doesn't have to be afraid that your relationship will change just because he prefers to date a different gender than what you may have expected. If your relationship was one in which things weren't spoken about so directly, you shouldn't feel pressure to now act differently. What your child wants is consistency—there is no reason why their sexuality should affect the fundamental ways that you interact with each other.

Remember that your child has the same brain and the same heart that they had before coming out to you. Sure, they might develop some new interests now that they are feeling more comfortable in their identity—but just because their taste in clothing, music, or activities may change, that doesn't undo the fact that they are still the same child whom you have known and loved for years. Allow yourself some room to readjust, to stumble, to hesitate in the wrong places, to say things in a way you didn't intend. This is part of adjusting to something new, and the more you work on communicating, the easier it will become. If you can't think of a good way to begin that journey, you have Kristin's complete permission to ask your child if they think that {insert current pop-star name} is a total babe.

Q: I accidentally found out that my child is gay. What do I do?

A: Accidentally finding out that your child is gay is sort of like discovering a birthday present two days before your birthday. You're stuck on the corner of "I know" and "but I'm not supposed to." Many parents, panicked, practice their I'm-so-surprised face in the mirror so that they won't hurt their child's feelings when they do decide to come out. While your child's sexuality isn't quite the same as a birthday present (though that would be an interesting gift to wrap), that feeling of knowing something that wasn't yet yours to know is always a tricky one to handle.

"A New Year's resolution to come out to my family"

I started gradually coming out to my friends when I was seventeen years old. Home was a different story, though. My dad would often say things like, "When you're older and have a nice boyfriend . . ." I felt really uncomfortable when moments like this happened because my answers were lies, and I'm the absolute worst liar in the world. That New Year's Eve, I made a resolution to come out to my family by the end of the year. I kept nearly telling them, and telling myself, "Today is the day!" but I'd never manage to get the words out. I knew they'd be totally fine with the idea, because they'd told my siblings and me that they didn't care who we fell in love with, as long as we found someone. So I couldn't figure out why it was so hard.

Things got worse when my celebrity crushes suddenly turned into a real crush on a woman I knew, and I wanted to talk about her all the time. I kept dropping her into the conversation when I recapped my days over family dinner. I knew she would never return my interest, and I wanted so badly to ask my mom for advice because she always gave relationship advice to my sisters. I couldn't, though, because I felt like I had to broach the "I'm gay" discussion first.

The year went on, and I started worrying that I was going to break my New Year's resolution. I always break my resolutions, but this was one I really wanted to achieve, and I knew I would hate myself for not doing it. When December arrived, I started panicking. With just a few weeks left, I wrote out huge, intricate plans for my coming-out speech, which even included rules for not using language that made me uncomfortable and a PowerPoint presentation. After I finished, I put it all in my drawer and thought about it every day, but I still couldn't bring myself to say the words.

Then it was New Year's Eve again, and I had just twelve hours left before the resolution would be broken. I found it impossibly hard to talk to my parents all day, because every conversation I had with them was followed by tears and the little voice in my head saying, "Tell them, tell them, tell them!" In the evening we settled down to watch TV. With every episode that went by, I was aware that it was another hour closer to midnight, and I still hadn't done it.

I quickly grabbed my computer and typed: "If I tell you who I have a crush on, do you promise not to make fun of me?" Then I held it for a while. My mouth was dry and I was sweatier than I had ever been before. It was ten minutes to midnight, and I thought I wasn't going to make it. Somehow, though, I managed to tell them to pause the program. I handed the computer over and my mom smiled and looked up at me and said, "Who do you have a crush on, then?" As fast as I could, I mumbled the names of three female leads from our favorite television shows. She replied immediately, "Of course. We all knew that already." My dad said he was proud of me. Then we went upstairs and watched the fireworks.

It was a little awkward for me afterward because I still had trouble admitting my feelings about people, and my mom just giggled whenever I mentioned liking anyone, which she hadn't done before. Eventually, though, we all adjusted. Now we spend time together chatting about who we like and what our "types" are, and my mom gives me advice just like she does with my sisters.

Shelly, 19

You may be overwhelmed by the information and not know where to turn, or be worried that the wrong approach might make your child feel backed into a corner. You may feel hurt that your child has been keeping something from you, or wonder if you did something to make them feel they couldn't talk to you.

If you are feeling railroaded by this information, try to take a few deep breaths. For many parents, this can be a large pill to swallow—it is completely normal for you to feel overwhelmed and a bit out to sea. It is important that you give yourself some time with the information before deciding how to proceed. Just as with many other things in life, impulse reactions are not always the best reactions, even when they are well-intentioned.

Also, recognize that your child's decision to keep this from you is not a reflection on your abilities as a parent. We receive countless letters from kids who know their parents will understand and accept them, but who still have a tough time finding the right words and the right moment to talk about their identity. In a lot of cases, this isn't something that they have clearly "known" for a long time, so working up the courage to talk about it can be difficult. Regardless of how you move forward with the information, you should try to trust that this "secret" is merely a part of their journey, not an indicator of a cataclysmic error on your part.

Your next steps depend on your relationship with your child. The information you stumbled upon might indicate that they very much *want* to talk about these things but are struggling with *how*—perhaps you overheard a phone conversation or discovered a note in which they specifically told a friend how scared they were to talk to you about their sexuality. If this is the case, you can absolutely help open that door and be honest with them about your accidental discovery.

If you decide to talk to your child directly:

✳ Make sure they know you weren't intentionally snooping. Keeping and maintaining trust is key.

✳ Tell them as many times as you feel is necessary that you love and support them.

✳ Don't say things like, "I don't care" or "It's not a big deal." This may be a very big deal for your child. Even if you are completely okay and unfazed by the information, they should know that you *do* care—in a positive way.

✳ Allow them their gut reaction. Maybe they will be angry at first, or maybe they won't want to talk about it further during this particular discussion. Let them know that there is no pressure to delve into things they aren't ready to talk about at this point, but you are always there to listen to them.

Your accidental discovery, however, might indicate that your child is still feeling very unsure about their sexuality or is not quite ready to talk to you about such things. Maybe you saw a love letter to a best friend or you found a personal blog where they are exploring some new feelings. If this is the case, then the best option is to tuck the information in the back of your brain and wait for them to approach you directly. It is important for your child to have space so they can understand their sexuality enough to communicate it clearly—when they are ready. In the interim, there are a few things you can do to help digest the information and prepare for that eventual conversation.

If you decide to wait until your child tells you:

* Make sure you have an outlet for your feelings. While you shouldn't go off and tell everyone in the neighborhood, it is absolutely okay to tell a trusted friend or two about your discovery. Just make sure those trusted few know this isn't common knowledge until your child is ready.

* Allow your child their continued privacy. You stumbled upon something accidentally, and now perhaps your interest is piqued and you want to know more. It will be difficult at times, but continuing to respect their privacy will only strengthen your relationship's ability to move forward.

* Drop small, supportive hints. This will foster an environment where your child will feel safe to eventually speak to you about their identity. This doesn't mean suddenly and unexpectedly putting a poster of Elton John over the dining room table, but you can certainly speak openly about human rights and current events!

* When your child does approach you, be honest. You don't have to pretend you never knew—unless you are a brilliant actor, they will likely pick up on the fact that you are not hearing this information for the first time. Explain to them that you accidentally came across something that made you think they were gay, but you wanted to give them the space they needed to initiate the conversation themselves.

* Read this book. Good job—you are already ahead of the curve.

For many, the coming-out process helps clarify and solidify the intricacies of their identity. The coming-out process is also just that: a process. Whether you decide to talk to your child immediately or wait for them to approach you, this won't be how either of you "expected" it to happen—and that is okay. Coming out is never how we imagine it might be, and it is never something that we are prepared for on either end of the dialogue. Whatever decision you make, remember that you will get many chances to work through your thoughts, your questions, and your emotions.

Q: **I think my child is gay, but they haven't come out to me yet. Should I ask them?**

My favorite pastime at the age of fifteen was to collect piles of Britney Spears memorabilia. My mother approached me one afternoon and, peering over my shoulder at the pictures of Britney, asked in her thick Southern accent, "Dan-yell, are you gay?" Now, if I had felt anything

toward Britney Spears other than a deep appreciation for her perfor-
mance abilities, the question might have opened up a much-needed con-
versation. The issue, though, was that I had absolutely no idea what she
was talking about—I wasn't gay! I had a huge crush on a boy at school and
was devastated daily that his interest was not returned. At that point, I
couldn't grasp why my mother had made this connection. It wasn't until
four years after this exchange that I began noticing an attraction to
other women.

—*Dannielle*

A: As a parent, you may simply have a gut feeling about your child. You may also have noticed a change in behavior, have seen something they posted online, or wondered about a relationship they have with a close friend. There is a chance that you are correct in your thinking, but there is also a chance that you are wrong. Even if you are right, you may be far ahead of your child's process. What's more, when you ask your child if they are gay, or imply it with prodding questions, it can result in them feeling judged, scrutinized, or visibly "different" from others—even if that isn't your intent.

An important part of the coming-out process is having the ability to communicate your identity to those closest to you, on your own terms. For this reason, it is often best to give your child the space they need to approach you when they feel most secure and comfortable in their own identity. Although Dannielle's mother was correct in her assumptions, her query made Dannielle worry that everyone else around her also thought she was gay. She also wondered what made her mother jump to that conclusion and started to feel exceptionally self-conscious about her behavior. No matter how gently the question is phrased or how supportive the intention, the implication is generally, "There is something about you that seems unlike others."

Also, be wary of trying to coax the information out of your child indirectly. Being questioned about how much time they might be spending with a certain friend will tip them off to the fact that you might have a bigger question lurking behind the decoys. Remember that you've been in this world for a considerably longer time, and exploring and understanding attraction and sexuality for the first time is a confusing experience. What is seemingly clear to you may take them a much longer time to understand. If your child is trying to work out their own confusions and also worrying about how and when to talk about those confusions with you, those not-so-subtle hints can make them feel angry, pressured, and further confused.

Gibson, who is seventeen and out to his family, thought the coming-out moment would be much easier if his parents would just ask him if he was gay. He figured it would circumvent the awkward moment of starting the conversation on his own. What he discovered, however, was that when his parents did ask him, he was so blindsided by the moment that he denied it! "In the end, I felt like it made it harder to tell them," he said, "because it seemed more like I had blatantly lied to them, instead of just having not explicitly told them about my sexuality." Asking your child can often cause a moment of panic—even if your tone is supportive and compassionate. In the moment, many kids will freeze and say what they may think you want to hear, which then leaves them in an even trickier position.

If you think that your child might be gay, the best approach is to create a safe and accepting environment. If your child *is* gay, this will help them work up the courage to talk with you once they better understand their own identity. Talk about current events in your home and voice your support for equality. Ask how kids are treating each other at school. Express your discontent with how cruel people can be to those who they think are "different" from themselves. You do not have to be gay or have a gay child to be vocal about human equality and respect for all individuals. The more you engage in dialogue around those and other issues, the more your child will understand that they have a loving parent who will accept them exactly as they are. This will allow them to feel safe, to explore and understand their own identity, and to approach you with their feelings when they are ready.

Q: **My child wants to come out at school, but I am concerned for their safety.**

A: We've been through a lot as a society to get to where we are today, but alongside the progress, many people are still made to feel inadequate based on a variety of qualities—sexuality among them. You have likely seen stories on television or in

"I'll always remember the day he told us."

———

Last October, my son Daniel told me and my wife that he's gay. I know the exact date—it was the first of October. We were having spaghetti and meatballs that night, and we haven't had spaghetti and meatballs in our house since—now it's a joke. Daniel said, "I want to tell you something that you probably already know. I'm gay." And then we asked the question that parents rarely know not to ask: "Are you sure?"

For me, it was a complete surprise. I was totally unprepared. I have several gay friends and employees, and I've never viewed them as different from anyone else. When it was in my own house, though, I didn't know how to handle it. I was in shock. I cried for two days—my tears were tears of pain for what I imagined Daniel was going through. But when I looked at him, I felt he was the same smart, happy kid.

After he told us, Daniel thought that we were going to kick him out of the house, that we wouldn't love him anymore, and that things were going to change. I think he was surprised when we didn't react the way he thought we would. We said, "We love you no matter what. You're our child." My wife's first call was to a psychologist friend of ours who has known Daniel since he was very little. My wife said, "Daniel just came out to us. What do we do? Where do we go?"

The one thing that helped me calm down was the support from my friends. I just told a couple of very close friends, because I felt like I needed to share this with somebody other than my wife. The resounding response was, "So what? He's Daniel. He's the same loving kid."

That gave me a lot of strength. And then, as more people heard, they would call me and say, "Hey, Sergio, I just found out. You know, Daniel is a great kid." There are definitely people out there who can be ignorant and closed-minded, but we live in a society where there is a lot more understanding, and I saw so much of it when it came to Daniel.

The first week after my son came out to us, I went to see a therapist, and I told him what I was going through. He told me point blank, "Sergio, you're doing everything right. You love your child." That meant a lot to me.

Now that I've had some time to process all of the things I was feeling when Daniel first came out, I find that I feel grateful. Grateful that my son was smart enough to have the nerve to come and tell us at this age, and that we get to know him completely as he grows older.

Sergio, 51

magazines that highlight some of the ways students bully each other, both in school and on the Internet, and you may be afraid that your child's identity will make them a target for bullying. That fear doesn't make you overbearing or silly or dramatic—it makes you a sweet, caring, excellent parent. The most important thing you can do with those fears is face them, examine them, and talk about them openly. This shouldn't be a you-against-your-child scenario; this should be an experience that you have *with* your child, in which you talk about your concerns and questions together.

The hardest fact to face may be that this is ultimately your child's decision. Even if you were to have brilliant, sound reasons for them to keep this a secret, there is simply no way to control what your child communicates to their friends or to the school community at large. You do, however, have every right to talk to them about your feelings or suggest that they look at all angles of the situation before they go forward with their choice. A great way to open this conversation is to say, "I'm concerned about you coming out at school and would really like to talk about a few things, but I know this is ultimately your decision to make, and I support you and stand behind you, always." This lets them know that you respect their ability to decide things on their own. That respect allows them to hear what you are saying much more clearly than if they thought you were trying to tell them what they should or shouldn't do. Asking questions is often much more powerful than making rules. The discussion you have will help them consider factors that may not have occurred to them, and it will also help you have a better understanding of the climate at their school.

Some questions you could ask include:

* How do you think the other kids at school will react?

* Do you have any friends who already know? What do they think?

* Are there any clubs or anything at your school like a Gay-Straight Alliance, where you can talk to others about your experience?

It may also help to talk to your child about their reasons for coming out at school. They might feel pressure in having to lie about their interests on a daily basis. Perhaps they have found a group of allies within their school and so they are now ready to take this step with the support that surrounds them. It may be that they want to change minds and be at the forefront of the activist community in your town. Those are all very valid and very different places to be coming from, and that information will help you to better understand the larger picture.

While asking questions can help you to better understand the surrounding circumstances and climate, you can also take an active role to help create a safer environment for your child and many others. Countless organizations exist explicitly to uproot bullying in schools. Several are listed in the Resources on page 222, and can provide further tools to help create a dialogue around these issues. There are films that can be shown in schools, curriculum that can be implemented, and meetings that can be organized to look at the specific issues facing the students in your community. Talk to your child about these resources, and ask if they would like you to become involved at their school. They may be thrilled that you have taken this interest, knowing that your voice will help them get administration and teachers to listen to their concerns. However, they may not be ready for you to be personally involved in a very active way. Hear them out and work to come up with a plan in which you both feel involved *and* comfortable.

Q: **I think my very young child might be gay. What should I do?**

A: Many parents of gay children say they "always knew." When asked how, some parents indicate that their child's choice in toys or dress was what informed them, others say they noticed a telling way that their child behaved around certain individuals, and many say that it was simply an inexplicable gut feeling.

First off, it's important to note that coming to conclusions based on behavior or interests can be complicated. A full discussion of gender and its relationship to sexuality is far too complex a knot to untie in just a few paragraphs (though we'll get into it more in chapter 7), but it is an important topic to look at briefly within this context. Is it true that little boys who like to play with dolls wind up having a preference for men later in life? Sure, sometimes. However, plenty of men who loved playing with dolls are attracted to women. There are some women who hated dresses, loved playing in the dirt, and are attracted to men. The combinations of outward gender expression and sexual attraction are endless. As you watch your child develop, keep in mind that an interest in certain toys or certain clothing does not necessarily reveal something about their orientation.

That said, for one reason or another, you may still suspect that your child is gay. Remember that there are (at least) two people involved in navigating this question: you and your child. Accordingly, there are certain things that you may want to do for yourself, and things that you will want to do for your child.

The best step you can take for yourself is to talk to others about your thoughts and questions. As with so many other things in the land of parenthood, discussing your experiences with people you trust and love will always help you better understand your feelings and make your path forward much clearer. No matter your child's sexuality, learning more about LGBTQ issues will better prepare you for answering future questions that they may have. Seek out resources within parent groups or LGBTQ groups such as Parents, Families and Friends of Lesbians and Gays (PFLAG), a U.S. nonprofit that acts as an ally advocacy organization as well as a support network for families and friends of LGBTQ people. See the Resources on page 222 for more information on support groups and literature. If in ten years your child is totally straight and you were completely wrong, the worst thing that you've done is familiarize yourself with a community different from your own. That is wonderful!

Where your child is concerned, the name of the game is support, inclusivity, and open dialogue. As we discussed earlier in this chapter, asking any child if they are gay—whether they are five or fifteen—can be very alienating. For a young child who may not completely understand what the word *gay* means, asking such a direct question can also be incredibly confusing. So, rather than confronting your child, show them support by making sure they know that, whoever they are, they will be loved unconditionally.

Here are a few simple steps you can take:

* Talk about the many different types of families in the world. You may have a home with a mom and a dad, but it is important to always let children know that there are homes that have just one mom, some that have two dads, and some that have a grandparent or a foster parent. See the Resources for a list of children's books that do a great job at illustrating these concepts.

* Explain things simply. Many people think that young children can't or shouldn't be told about being gay because they won't understand or because they shouldn't be learning about sex. Your children know that boys love girls at this age, so it is completely reasonable that they know (and can understand)

that boys sometimes love boys, and girls sometimes love girls as well. They will probably receive this information exactly as they received the rest of the information out there, with a shrug and a few questions. Your telling them that sometimes boys love other boys does not have to include an advanced talk about sex of any kind.

* Allow them to dress and play how they choose. Children should never be told that certain games or toys are "only for boys" or "just for girls." This creates rigid structures of gender to which hardly any of us can conform, regardless of our sexuality, and it can lead to them feeling like the things they enjoy are inherently wrong or bad.

* Be honest about the actions of others. When you allow your child to dress and play how they choose, there is a chance that their peers will make fun of them for being different. If this happens, explain to your child that some people don't like when others are different from them, but that you will support them, always. Let them talk to you about the things they are feeling, and navigate those experiences together as a team.

These few simple steps will create an open environment in which your child will be able to explore and play without feeling that their parent thinks they are "wrong" or "bad." Children's interests and behaviors change often when they are at such a young age, which is why it is so difficult to ever really *know* anything concretely about who they will grow up to be. All children come to understand attraction and sexuality at different points in their development, which is why allowing them freedom to express the things they desire and play with the toys they love—as well as encouraging an awareness of many different identities—will help them to understand themselves better.

THE BOTTOM LINE

* It's likely that your child has only recently come to understand that they are gay—so working up the courage to talk about it can sometimes be scary! Be patient and supportive so they feel comfortable talking to you when they're ready.

* Work at creating a home environment that is safe and accepting of all identities, all the time.

* Be as consistent in your parenting style as possible—there is no reason why your kid's sexuality should alter fundamental ways in which you interact with each other.

* Allow young children to express themselves and play with the toys that they prefer. Give them tools to understand the world in colors that are not only pink and blue.

CHAPTER 2: **First Reactions**

After the dust has settled on the initial "I'm gay" announcement, you will likely have a whole host of questions banging around inside your brain. You may be afraid your child will face discrimination, never get married, or feel out of place in the world at large. Many of these worries may have arisen regardless of your child's sexuality, but given this new context, things may seem more overwhelming. Know that you are equipped to handle these concerns and questions, and that there are resources around you that can help.

Don't be afraid to ask questions. The more information you gather, the easier it will be to navigate these new surroundings. Ask your child, ask your friends, and seek out books, articles, and support groups that can help you better understand your child and this process as a whole. Take the time you need to reflect; you can't get all of the answers you seek in just a few short weeks or months. The fact that you are beginning this journey by seeking out resources and answers is a clear indicator of how much you love your child, and how much you want to be able to understand and support them.

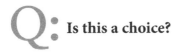

Q: Is this a choice?

Personally, I don't feel as though I was born gay. I also don't feel as though I explicitly chose my sexuality. I feel that I came to understand myself, my attractions, and my interests based on a ton of factors—some that felt more inherent to my person, and others that I found in the world around me. I know that I didn't choose whom to have crushes on or fall in love with, but I have also never felt as though "I always knew." What I do know is that, given the choice today, I would choose this life—my sexuality included. I love my life and I love the way I view the world around me because of who I am and whom I love. I think we all come to understand our sexualities in our own unique ways.

—Kristin

A: It is important to be cautious when talking about sexuality as something that is or is not a "choice." That word—*choice*—is a very narrow way of describing a complex experience. When we hear that someone "chooses" something, we think in simple terms: choosing a red shirt over a green one or choosing french fries over a salad. That is not an accurate way to frame our experience of sexuality or attraction. Think, for a moment, about your own sexuality. If you identify as "straight," do you feel as though you made a conscious choice to feel that way? Did you wake up one day, look at the various options presented to you, and say, "You know, straight seems like the identity I prefer, so I will pick that one," and then suddenly, after choosing, find yourself attracted to a particular gender? Probably not. It is never as simple as picking an identity out of a bucket and having that choice or decision inform your desires and interests. If this is what we mean when we say "choice," then no, sexuality is certainly not something that any of us choose. However, it is very important to reflect on what you mean when you ask this question. For some, it is simple curiosity; given only your own experience with sexuality, you might wonder how someone comes to understand themselves as something other than heterosexual. For others, it is a question that actually means, "Can I help my kid change this part about them?" or "Did my kid decide to be gay?"

For those who are curious as to the experience itself: Every person has their own, personal relationship with sexuality. There are individuals who feel they have known they were gay since the moment they could form a memory, who feel this is in their DNA, and that they were, quite literally, "born this way." There are others who came to understand their sexuality at a later stage in their life, and who believe that part of their desires and attractions were informed by experiences they had with the world around them. Still others feel they are somewhere in the middle—that part of their identity was always hardwired, but different experiences and interactions also helped to shape and foster their attractions. There is simply no way to sift through the complex brain maze that determines and directs desires and end with one final answer on how it all works, because it is different for all of us. The only way to understand your kid's experience with sexuality is to ask them. You may find out that they have known since they were three years old, or that they didn't think much about it until this year, but regardless of how they have come to understand themselves, that understanding is valid, real, and true.

For those who want to know if sexuality is a decision or something that can be changed: no, it is not; and no, it cannot. As we discussed previously, reflecting on your own experience with sexuality is an incredible way to get a better sense of how complicated and intricate that understanding can be. Just as you cannot change the way your brain and heart and body interact with the people and the world around you, neither can your child. Trying to deny any part of who you are—sexually or otherwise—is troublesome, isolating, and damaging. Whenever we try to refuse any part of ourselves, that part grows and demands that we give it the attention it is due. Your kid is your kid, all parts, all desires, all attractions included.

Q: Is this my fault?

A: *Fault* is another tricky word. The question, "Who is to blame?" implies that there is something inherently wrong with your child's sexuality. Therefore, the first step in looking at this question is to phrase it in a way that will allow for a more open-ended discussion. This isn't (or at least, shouldn't be) about pointing a judging finger at yourself or someone else; this is about you wondering *why* your child's sexuality is different from your own, or different from what you may have anticipated.

As we discussed in the previous question, coming to understand personal sexuality is a different process for everyone, and it doesn't hinge on any one moment or a simple "decision." There is no way for anyone to boil down their attractions and desires to one specific origin. And truthfully, even if we could whittle down all of the layers and find out that, *yes, at age three when you told your daughter she had to go to ballet, that somehow informed and shaped her future sexuality*, what would you do with that information? Knowing *why* your kid is gay won't make you any better of a parent. What's more important is accepting and supporting your child.

It is okay to open up a dialogue around some of these questions, so long as you are able to speak in a way that will not make your kid feel that who they are is a bad thing. Don't approach the topic by saying things like, "Are you like this because of me?" or "Did I do something wrong to make you this way?" Rather, frame

This Is a Book for Parents of Gay Kids

the conversation in a positive way by saying something like, "I would love to talk more about when you started to understand this part of yourself. Do you think this was something that you've always felt, or do you think experiences in your life shaped you?" If your child is able to talk openly about these things, you will be able to learn more about how they view their identity. This may help you let go of some of the guilt you are feeling. If your child is not yet ready to answer these questions, have patience. They will eventually get to a place where you can have more open communication. For now, focus on the positive aspects of your child's life (their sexuality included!), and remember that people don't single-handedly create and inform the desires of others.

Q: I think this is just a phase.

A: Most of us go through different stages in life regarding a variety of topics—sexuality included. Just as our tastes in food and music may change over our lifetime, we also evolve in terms of whom we are attracted to and why we are attracted to them based on an array of factors, such as appearance, personality, interests, and sometimes gender. We change, we grow, and maybe your child *is* unsure—but maybe they are as sure as anything they have ever known. Their sexuality may remain consistent throughout their lives, or it may vary, but this doesn't make their current identity less valid. Every kid—in fact, every *person*—has a different

"What did I do wrong?"

⸻

When my daughter came out to me at the age of twenty-five, I felt overwhelmed with emotion. As a mother, my mind quickly went to, "How could I not see this? What did I miss? What did I do wrong?" Instead of making it all about her, I made it all about me and my abilities as a parent. I searched for a reason for it not to be true. This was not the life I wanted for my daughter. I wanted the son-in-law and the grandkids. You know—the traditional life. I also knew that she was anything but traditional.

Since my daughter lived in a different city when she came out, she told me over the phone. This was not ideal, but probably worked best due to the high emotions we were both experiencing. After a tearful phone conversation, I ran to her childhood bedroom, thinking that somehow it would make me feel closer to her. I thought maybe some clue of information would be revealed that would help me get my head around this new information.

I pulled out old pictures of her in school, yearbooks, journals, anything I could find to see what I'd missed. Surely I had missed something. A perfect mom would have recognized this early, or would have raised her in a better environment where she could have felt more comfortable and discovered this earlier. Looking back at all of her struggles in high school and college, my emotions shifted from wishing she wasn't gay to blaming myself for not allowing her to be who she truly was. She had been acting as the person I had wanted her to be, instead of finding herself. I had always harshly judged parents who lived vicariously through their children; now I was coming to the realization that I, too, was guilty of this.

I do not like emotional pain, and I try to find the quickest path through it. My husband says that I can leap to new paradigms much quicker than most people. It only took me a couple of days to realize that what I really needed to be focused on was not what I did or didn't do in her childhood. That was in the past and couldn't be changed. What mattered most now was what I was doing today. What mattered most was what my child needed right now: my unconditional love. I could sort things out later—if they even needed to be sorted out. A mother never wants to see her child in pain. My child was going through the most painful experience of her life, afraid she would lose our relationship because of being herself. She needed assurance that I would be there, no matter what.

I so badly wanted to jump on a plane, run to her, and scoop her up like she was three years old again, hold her, and tell her everything would be all right. Instead, we had long phone conversations, fraught with more tears and emotion. She knew, though, through these conversations, that I would continue to stand by her no matter what.

I'm proud of her, and I'm extremely proud to be her mother.

Lynn, 51

journey when it comes to sexuality. What matters is who they are and how they feel *right now*. As a parent, you probably know how many unexpected things crossed your path over the course of your lifetime. The same will happen to your child. Do your best to remain flexible in moving along with your child's experience instead of trying to anticipate the future.

J, who came out to her parents when she was sixteen, said that her mom would address her sexuality by saying things like, "Oh well, it's because you're questioning right now," or "You're just confused." These words upset her, and made her feel disrespected because, as she put it, "I had started questioning when I was about thirteen, so by the time I was sixteen and telling people I was gay, it was because I knew I was gay. It was my identity." Respecting your child's identity is possible, even if you wonder if it will remain consistent over time. Even if everything on your insides is screaming, "But I know this isn't true," fighting your child on how they identify is often counterproductive. The more you insist that they are *not* what they say they are, the more likely they are to devote their efforts to proving you wrong instead of focusing on their own process of personal reflection.

Allow your child to experience their own journey; let them make mistakes, get bad haircuts, fall in love. You've had a front row seat to their development for many years, so it may be a challenge to concede that you didn't anticipate this particular facet of their identity. Do your best to appreciate who they are, and how they identify, right now. When it comes down to it, your kid might have markedly different interests in two or five or ten or twenty years. Perhaps you're right and they will explore their attractions and come to a different understanding than they currently have. However, you could also be wrong. Your child, in having the freedom to explore who they are, may meet someone of the same gender, fall madly in love, and grow old with them, happier than you could have ever imagined.

Q: Am I allowed to ask questions?

There was a time when my dad's questions about my life (whether in regard to love, friends, or politics) would embarrass me horribly. It wasn't that I didn't love my dad or want him to know about my life—it was just because I didn't yet know how to talk about the things I was feeling. He never stopped asking, though, and if he saw that I was a bit uncomfortable he would just laugh a little and say, "We don't have to talk about this, Daughter, I just like knowing what's going on with you." It took a few years before I learned how to have some of these conversations with my dad without turning bright red, but I was never upset that he was trying. In fact, I valued it enormously. Now that I'm a bit older, I talk to my dad about everything. He's always the first to know what's going on in my life, who I'm dating, how my friends are doing, what political issue is upsetting me at the moment. He and I are closer than ever, and I'm convinced it's because he never stopped asking questions.

—Dannielle

"My mom said I was too girly to be gay."

My mother takes the most beautiful photographs. Because of her profession, I can glimpse, in some small way, how she perceives the world. This has been a gift into understanding her as a person. But this is not a story about my mother's photography. This is a story about finally seeing what my mother saw when I was seventeen.

During the latter part of my time in high school, I insisted I was going to the U.S. Naval Academy. I was going to major in chemistry, become a cargo pilot, and later be an astronaut. I spent hours reading about NASA, I went to a camp about science and technology in public policy, and I became president of my high school chemistry club. My mother, who had dated midshipmen before, was heartsick at the idea of me at the Naval Academy. A soft-spoken, sensitive child who liked poetry and cried easily—surely these were not the makings of a naval officer. Looking back, my mother worried that the Navy would crush me. I was hoping that the Navy would make me strong.

I needed strength because I feared that if anyone knew I was attracted to other girls, I would be reviled. Finally, one evening after dinner, my mother questioned me about an e-mail I'd received from a friend. I admitted to her what I feared most—that I was a lesbian. Our initial conversation was reasonably calm, but she assured me that what I was going through was a phase. Women are attractive to look at, she pointed out, and I shouldn't mistake attraction for simply enjoying beauty in other people. Our family had endured a year of my grandparents being extremely ill, and I was probably reacting to the stress. Besides, I was so girly, and had always been girly—my mother joked that she was more of a lesbian than I was, because she was very athletic and a dedicated tennis player in her youth. I loved doing my hair, makeup, and nails—what part of that said *lesbian*? She asked me if I was given the choice between dating a boy and dating a girl, all things equal, which would I choose? Meekly, I muttered that I would choose the girl. My mother thought I was just saying that to save face. Our talk drew to a close, and I begged her not to tell my father.

Over the next few weeks, my mother made comments about the masculine appearance of the female astronauts I so admired. She had previously joked about me having a crush on a good female friend of mine (I did); after our conversation, those jokes ceased. I withdrew. I hid my secret, cut ties with my one friend to whom I had come out, and went away to a liberal arts college. I was miserable my freshman year. I kept trying to balance my mother's opinion that I was going through a phase with my own feelings. I had no idea which to trust; in the past, my mother had always been right. She had my best interests at heart in my childhood, and her intuition has an irritating way of usually being correct. How could she be wrong now? I drifted away from chemistry and became a French major instead. I was girly—maybe this was a field that suited me better. I dated a few men in college, briefly, but I was recognizing that the butterflies-in-the-stomach sort of feeling only happened with my female crushes.

I spoke with my parents many times during that first year of college. We spoke over the phone because I lived two hours away in a larger city. My mother grew angry when she found out that I had gone to a gay club with some friends (why I'd even told her, I'm not certain). She had looked the club up on the Internet and told me that the people in the photos looked like "freaks." In retrospect, her "freaks" comment might have been the best thing she could have ever said. Though it hurt, deeply, it also caused me to grow angry. Through my anger, I was able to question her judgment and evaluate whether or not her opinion was in keeping with what I knew to be true. She told me that no boys at work would ask me out with my hair that short, and if I kept acting like a lesbian, everyone was going to treat me like one. In reality, frustratingly, not one woman approached me, but the haircut gave me a confidence I'd never had before.

Somehow my mother and I moved through all of the hurt together. After a lot of tears, and a lot of talking, eventually something seemed to click. As for me, I carried my anger far beyond its usefulness. It was only after examining my frustration through therapy that I began to see the way out. I expressed annoyance that my mother didn't even remember half the hurtful things she'd said, and my therapist told me, "Your mother has worked very hard to get to the place where she is now. She deserves some credit for that." Initially, that, too, made me angry, then indignant, and then I finally accepted its truth. I realized my mother didn't recall saying hurtful things because she never meant the things she said to be perceived as hurtful.

My mother has been supportive all along. Even when she used language that wounded me, she loved me. Hoping that this was all a phase was another way of trying to protect me—just like she wanted to protect me from the hardships of being in the Navy. What matters is that I love my mother more each day, and she loves me, too. My mother took a photograph of me recently. I hate most photographs of myself, but I love this one. I look beautiful seen through her eyes—a small glimpse into how much she loves me. It is my mother, after all, who gave me the courage to go my own way.

Molly, 26

A: Not only are you allowed to ask questions, you are encouraged to do so. Asking your child questions means that you care about them and that you want to better understand them, and these are markers of a wonderful parent. Of course, these efforts may not be rewarded immediately, and perhaps your child will express embarrassment or even annoyance at what they perceive to be an intrusion into their personal life. Here's the thing to remember: It is possible to communicate how you are feeling, express the reasons that you want to better understand their feelings, and *also* give your child the space they may need as they come to better understand themselves. They may not be immediately receptive, but over time they'll come to appreciate your interest.

A great place to start is by simply telling them that you have questions and would like to talk about them. You can say, "Do you mind if I ask you questions?" or "Is it okay if we talk about a few things?" You can also make the initial conversation a bit more specific. You might ask, "I was wondering if you would be comfortable telling me more about how you came to realize that you were gay? It would really help me to better understand things." You may find that your child is excited to share more about this with you and that this sparks an incredible dialogue. If it does, fantastic. If it doesn't, persevere and try again another time. Have patience with yourself and your child within those discussions, because this is new territory for you both. When the conversation ends, be clear with your child that they can always talk to you and approach you with any questions they might have—they *will* have questions, and leaving the door open will create more opportunities for communication.

If you receive a reaction that is tinged with embarrassment, annoyance, exasperation, or hesitation, that is also okay! This just means that your child is partway through the process of becoming comfortable in their own skin, and conversing about certain things may not feel quite right just yet. Oluremi, who came out to her parents at age sixteen, reflected on her experience with her parents' questions, saying, "I always thought it was okay for them to ask questions, but I didn't always know how or feel ready to answer them." If your child isn't in a place to answer your questions, just say something along the lines of, "It is okay for us to not talk about this right now. I just want you to know that I care about you and that it will help me to better understand certain things once you are ready to have these conversations." Wait a few months, and then try the same approach—ask them if they are feeling more able to talk about things with you, and see if things have shifted.

If your child isn't quite ready to talk, it is still very important to deal with your unanswered questions. There are thousands of parents out there who have had similar questions and experiences— it is just a matter of getting in touch with the right groups and communities (see the Resources on page 222 for more). You can learn and go through this process on your own terms while your child becomes more comfortable with who they are. It is more than likely that, given some time, it will become easier for you to ask questions and easier for your child to answer them.

Q: Will my other kids be gay?

A: It's possible, but it's not something that anyone can predict!

There are plenty of siblings out there with very diverse sexualities. Just as one of your children may be more interested in sports, while another is exceptionally talented at singing, your children can be very different when it comes to sexuality. We could talk for hours about the biology of it all, and whether having one gay child does, in fact, make it more likely for your other children to be gay. But none of the science behind these claims is concrete, and there's absolutely no way to determine if your other kids will be gay based on the sexuality of *one* of your children.

We have spoken to several parents who are worried that if their other kids know that their sibling is gay, they will have more reason to be gay themselves. This is, quite simply, not how things work when it comes to our sexual identities. Try to think about how you would have felt about your own sexuality if your sibling had been gay, or if a very close friend of yours had come out to you in middle school or high school. Do you think that this would have changed your identity? Perhaps, if you had already been curious, you would have felt more confident in exploring your sexuality or speaking about it. However, that knowledge would not have changed the fundamentals that inform and create your sexuality. We will talk about this more in the following chapters, but the bottom line is this: Being honest with your other children will not alter their personal desires and interests. Your children are who they are, period.

What's more, being open about and accepting toward all identities (both within and outside of your family unit) can make all the difference if it turns out that another one of your kids *is* gay. Coming out tends to be a much harder process for a child when they have a sibling who is already out to the family. We have spoken to many kids who have watched a sibling come out to their parents, and who are terrified to come out themselves because this will mean that now *two* of their parents' children are gay. Many kids feel that this will push their parents over an edge of some kind, and that what was once acceptance will turn into disappointment, anger, or sadness. They also fear their coming out will be seen as less valid, as a possible "copycat" move, or a means of just wanting to be like their sibling.

For these reasons alone, it is so important that your support of your "out" kid is seen and heard by your other children. As we already discussed, this support will not change who they are, but it will help them to better understand themselves and to share those findings with you. If you are a parent of more than one child, and you speak about how you are "so glad" that your other children "aren't gay," this can (and likely will) close all doors of communication. Make sure to voice your support around your other children, and also strive to use inclusive language. If you ask them a question about dating, phrase the question in an inclusive way. Rather than saying to your son, "Are you interested in any girls at school?" ask, "Are there any people who you are dating or interested in?" This is not only sensitive to them, but it also shows respect and support for the child who has come out to you.

The name of the game is treating all of your children equally, and with respect. Some families do have more than one child who is gay; other families have six children in which only one child is gay. There is no way to "know" about the intricacies of your other children based on the qualities of one child. It is, however, possible for your support and honesty to allow for all of your kids to feel confident expressing themselves, no matter who they are.

THE BOTTOM LINE

* Using the word *choice* when talking about sexuality can be problematic. No one chooses sexuality like they choose a dressing for their salad, but for many it is not as simple as just being "born that way."

* No one person single-handedly creates or informs another person's sexuality. Try to focus on the positive instead of trying to understand the "cause."

* Allow your kid the space to explore their identity. Their understanding of themselves may remain consistent, or it may fluctuate, but that doesn't invalidate how they feel at this moment.

* Ask questions, and be patient if you don't receive a positive response immediately. Revisit your questions, and seek support from others who are in similar positions.

* The sexuality of one of your children does not and cannot determine the sexuality of any of your other children.

CHAPTER 3: Telling Others

While your child has to navigate the coming-out process, you, too, will be faced with decisions about sharing this information with people in your life. There are many factors to consider—among them, your own comfort level and your child's readiness to share this part of themselves with others. You may worry about whom to tell, or how to tell them, and the responses that you will receive from people close to you. Your child is not the only person who will have to come out to others; you will also have to make decisions about coming out as a parent of a gay child.

We all share information differently. There is no obligation for you to tell every person who crosses your path that you have a gay child, but you certainly can! Remember that the decision to tell others is personal and specific to you and your kid.

=====

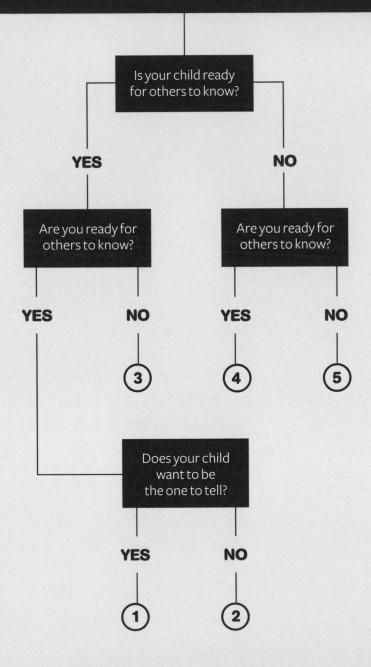

WHEN SHOULD I TELL PEOPLE?

Is your child ready for others to know?

YES

NO

Are you ready for others to know?

Are you ready for others to know?

YES

NO

YES

NO

③

④

⑤

Does your child want to be the one to tell?

YES

NO

①

②

Q: When should I tell people?

A: Telling others—whether it be family, friends, coworkers, or acquaintances—is something that happens at different times, depending on when you or your child are ready for that information to be shared. Since there are many permutations when it comes to telling others, we have created a chart to help guide you.

(1) You and your child both want others to know, and your child would prefer to be the one to tell others. Well, fantastic! This means your child is taking ownership of the experience, and since they are communicating something that is very personal to them, they'd like it to be done in their own words. The best thing you can do in this scenario is allow them the time and the space to tell others as they see fit, and let them know you are there for them if they ever want to talk about any of those experiences. Also, feel free to ask your child to keep you in the loop as things progress. If you think that certain individuals might have a harder time than others, you can absolutely have that discussion with your child beforehand. People will often surprise you and respond differently than you anticipate, but it is okay to tell your child that Aunt Becky might direct them to certain Bible passages or express less-than-positive religious views. This will give your kid a heads up, and may also inspire them to come out to that particular family member in a different way, or with more materials at the ready. (For more on coming out to religious friends and family, you can turn to chapter 6.)

(2) **You and your child both want others to know, and your child wants you to be the one to tell them.** This also makes a lot of sense. Your child is comfortable with who they are, but they are not yet experienced in having these conversations with relatives or family friends. They are looking to you because they need your help in tackling the task at hand. The best thing you can do in this scenario is talk to your child about what they would like you to communicate, specifically. It may be that they just need you to have that very first exchange in which all you say is, "Uncle Don, Lisa came out to us as a lesbian." You can field questions in the initial back and forth, but your child will likely be much more confident answering follow-up questions once the proverbial cat is out of the bag. There may be specific words they would like you to use, and you might need more clarity on what certain things mean, so just make sure they are clear with you so that you can be clear with others! Also, look at the "What will people think?" question in this chapter, which goes over specifics on actually having the my-kid-is-gay talk with others.

(3) **Your child wants everyone to know, but you are not yet ready to tell others.** You may still be dealing with your kid's coming-out moment yourself and need time to process that before sharing the news with others. That is a completely valid, totally understandable response. Your child has spent considerable time coming to understand themselves, but this is brand new for you and, as such, you may need some time to explore your feelings. Ultimately, this is your child's decision to make—but asking for some time to ready yourself for those conversations is understandable. Explain to your child that you just need a little time to talk more with them and to understand things a bit better. It may be helpful to give them an idea of a timeline, so that you both are aware of when you can revisit the discussion. For example, you can say, "I absolutely respect that you would like others in our family circle to know about this, and I am happy that you are feeling comfortable and ready to have that conversation. Since this is brand-new information for me, I would love if you could give me some time to digest it and also ask some more questions. I would love to be feeling a little more confident as well when family and friends talk to me about everything. How about we sit down and talk about this again three weeks from today, and go from there? Does that sound reasonable?" If this is agreeable to them, do make sure that this is only a short, transitional phase. Keeping your kid closeted for any substantial amount of time can be extremely detrimental to their well-being, as it creates an environment in which they feel they have to lie about themselves to people close to them.

(4) **You would like others to know, but your child doesn't feel ready.** In this scenario, your child doesn't yet feel comfortable with other people knowing about their sexuality, and they have come to you first with the information. Coming out is a huge step for a child (or anyone), and being able to have some control over who knows, and how they find out, is very important. If your child isn't ready for others to know just yet, you should respect those wishes. This is a journey for you both, but at this moment it is your child's process that should be put first. Allow them some time to navigate how it feels to be out to themselves and out to you before pushing them to tell others, or telling others on your terms. Revisit the discussion in a month or two, and check in to see how they are feeling at that point.

(5) **You and your child are both hesitant about telling others.** Given this combination, it is important to remember that you should not feel obligated to tell people. It is not the responsibility of anyone in the LGBTQ community to be vocal about their identity—this is a personal choice and it can vary. Right now, this is between you and your child, and that relationship is most important. Support your child and try to talk about the things that are making you both feel hesitant. The more comfortable you become talking to your child, the more comfortable you'll both be with the idea of telling others, should that be something that you'd like to do down the line.

"I didn't know how to tell my friends."

Zoe came out to me when she was eighteen years old. Up until that moment, we always had a good routine when it came to conversations—she'd tell me she wanted to talk about something and ask if it was a good time, I'd tell her I had to finish a couple of phone calls, and then we'd settle down to talk about what was on her mind. This particular night, though, I was lying in my bed not feeling so well, and in comes Zoe. She lays across me and says, "Mom, I have to tell you something." I was like, "Really? You have to tell me now?" She was adamant. "Yes, I have to tell you now." So, she did. She told me she was gay.

When it came to telling other people about Zoe's sexuality, we mostly didn't. I felt that, since nobody calls other people just to say, "My kid's a heterosexual," why should I call and make an announcement about my daughter? I didn't think it was anybody else's business, unless Zoe wanted them to know. But, of course, as with everything else, things were a little more complicated than they initially seemed.

A few months passed, and we were asked to go to dinner by our close friends—friends who have always adored Zoe. I told them that Zoe was going to be coming home from college that day, and they were thrilled and told us to bring her along. The complication was that Zoe was coming home with her girlfriend, Madi—and I didn't know how to explain that to my friends. Instead of trying to find the right words, I simply said, "Well, Zoe is bringing a friend with her." They, of course, immediately extended an invitation to her "friend."

I told Zoe the day she was headed home that she and Madi were invited to join us all for dinner, but then explained that I hadn't told our friends that the two of them were dating. Zoe drew a line in the sand. She said she wouldn't go to dinner unless everyone knew that she and Madi were a couple. She didn't want to lie. It made sense, and it was the first time Zoe had ever put her foot down about anything, but we had just a short amount of time before we had to leave. I didn't know what to do. My husband suggested that we just tell our friends that Zoe missed the train, so that we could avoid the conversation entirely. At that point, our extended family didn't even know. I had no idea what to expect. So, Zoe stayed home.

We went to dinner, and my friends, of course, said how they were so sorry that Zoe had missed the train. In that moment, I just couldn't lie. I told them, then and there. I said, "Well, actually, Zoe did not miss the train. Zoe's at home. She wants me to tell you that she's gay, and that her friend is not just her friend, her friend is her partner. I want you to know, too." They did not miss a beat. They asked me if she was happy, and I told them she was—she was really happy. The wife replied, "That's what's most important." Her husband said to me before we left dinner that night, "I want you to tell Zoe that she will always be a daughter to me and I expect her to be at dinner next time."

Michele, 58

Q: Whom should I tell? Their siblings? Their grand-parents? Our mailman?

When I came out to my parents, I was seventeen. My sister, Alyson, was twelve. My mom felt very strongly that Alyson was "too young to know," and that having a gay sister might somehow influence her understanding of her own sexuality. In simplest terms, my mom didn't want me to turn my sister gay. I didn't agree with that reasoning, but at the time I felt that I should do whatever I could to stay in my mom's good graces, so I obliged. I told my sister about three years later, when she was fifteen. She, as I expected, shrugged and moved along to bigger and better topics of conversation such as the origin of dinosaurs and the details of Einstein's biography (she really likes science), and our relationship has never wavered. There was not a moment in her life when she viewed my sexuality as something that would impact her own. She identifies as straight, likes boys, loves boys, and dates boys— just as she always has. In retrospect, I wish that I had told her along with the rest of my family, because I knew then that she wasn't "too young." I'm her sister, and this is a part of who I am.

—Kristin

A: If your child is in a place where they feel comfortable with you speaking to other people about their identity, deciding *whom* you should tell can be a bit overwhelming. Know that you are under no obligation to tell each and every person in your life that your child is gay. You certainly weren't walking around saying things like, "Hey, just so you know, John is heterosexual,"

before your son came out to you. The same goes for having a gay child. There is no need to make a general announcement about these things unless you want to or there is an explicit reason to do so.

Generally, the people you will want to tell outright are the people whom you hold dear, and who have been in your life for a long time. Since these are also the people you're likely to look to as sounding boards on personal matters, you can talk with them as openly as you always have. Telling your closest friends will enable you to talk about your thoughts on your daughter's new girlfriend just as you would have if she had been dating a boy. When it comes to those outside of your main circle of friends and family, whom you tell is more of a case-by-case basis. If you live in a rather conservative area, you may decide to remain a bit private with your personal affairs. This, however, is not always the case. Different people walk different paths, and so long as you are doing what makes you and your child feel centered and supported, you are doing the right thing. There is no need to go as far as to tell the mailman, but if you are proud of your child and happen to be wearing a gay pride T-shirt when your mail is delivered, you can definitely explain why!

Because there are many different groups of people with whom you may (or may not) want to share this information, we have elaborated on the next few pages.

THE SIBLINGS

Oftentimes, it will be your child's decision to tell their siblings just as they told you—when they are ready, and in their own words. However, there are some instances when *you* may be asked to tell your other children. Your child may prefer that you be the one to speak the initial words, if they are having a hard time finding the right moment. They might look to you to facilitate the conversation, or help them along in initiating that first exchange. Your child may also be out of your home, away at college or elsewhere, while their younger sibling or siblings are still at home with you.

If your child has simply asked that you initiate the conversation with their sibling for them, then you can (and should) tell your other kids. This will take different shapes depending on your personal (and varied) relationship with your other children. In talking to them, make sure to explain why you are the one telling them, that you support and love all your kids, and that they can come to you or their sibling with any questions they have.

You might also be questioning whether you should tell your other children because you are concerned about their age, and think they might be too young to fully understand. Kids are never too young to understand differences among people—if anything, they are much better equipped than those who have had a lifetime of learning what is "right" and "wrong" from the world around them. Children have much more flexibility in understanding that it is possible for people to love each other in combinations that are not only boys and girls. Explain things simply. *John likes boys the same way that Daddy likes Mommy* is enough to communicate the message. Most young children will respond with a question or two and then ask if they can watch television. There are several children's books listed in the Resources on page 222 that can help you facilitate these discussions.

THE GRANDPARENTS (AND OTHER FAMILY MEMBERS)

Telling your parents, or your spouse's parents, can often be a complicated issue to navigate. If the grandparents are in good health, then the decision to tell them will hinge on the same (or similar) factors that exist for the rest of the family. Telling extended family is different for everyone. It may happen all at once, or it may happen gradually over time. You may feel that speaking to your parents is the very first conversation you want to have, or you may be hesitant for a variety of reasons.

Michele, whose daughter Zoe came out to her as a lesbian when she was eighteen, had an extremely hard time when it came to telling her parents. She felt as though, in some way, her daughter being gay would make her own mother and father think less of her as a parent. She thought they might view Zoe's sexuality as a consequence of not being nurtured enough by Michele. "It took me a while to move past that, because I felt that I was a disappointment to them," she said. When Michele asked her parents what their thoughts were on Zoe's sexuality, they confessed that they hadn't known how to respond because

Michele had been crying when she delivered the news. Michele's parents had just wanted to be supportive of *their* daughter, and in doing so, hadn't had the chance in that first exchange to express their support of their granddaughter.

Many families also struggle with telling grandparents because of age or health conditions. They don't want to withhold information, but at the same time, they know that it might cause unnecessary stress, or be very confusing in the context of an aging person's experience. If not telling them is making you or your kid feel like you're constantly hiding something, then telling them is likely the right move. If you both feel you can share most other things about your lives, but that telling them will unnecessarily add to their stress or existing health issues, then the better decision may be to keep that information to yourselves. You and your child know your family better than anyone else, and so you will have to use that knowledge to help make the final decision. Weigh all the factors, and try to choose whichever option will bring you and your child the most peace of mind. There are no "wrong" answers here.

THE COWORKERS

When it comes to speaking with coworkers, or anyone else you see on a fairly regular (but not necessarily personal) basis, each decision you make will be different. You may find that each time you pass your boss's desk, you are being asked, "So, how is your son? Does he have a girlfriend?" Questions such as this one might make you uneasy and cause you to mumble a quick noncommittal answer under your breath, or may act as a wonderful impetus for you to say, "No, actually, my son doesn't date girls, but as soon as he has a boyfriend, I will let you know!" That interaction closely mirrors many moments that your child has on a daily basis with others—and can give you insight into how complicated those coming-out moments can be.

If you feel comfortable talking openly about your kid's sexuality, then you should answer those kinds of questions honestly. Generally speaking, it is easiest to come out as a parent of a gay child when the conversation meanders to that topic on its own, rather than just standing up at your desk and shouting, "I have a gay kid!" It may be, though, that being completely open at your place of employment is not realistic for you, or not what you would prefer. You may be concerned about the repercussions of making your child's sexuality common knowledge. You may just prefer to keep your personal life to yourself at your workplace. Just like all else, this is ultimately a decision for you and your kid to navigate together. If you are hesitant about telling your coworkers, make sure that you explain this clearly to your child. Ensure that they know you are not keeping this a secret because you are ashamed of them in any way, but because you are concerned that the response of others might make for a negative work environment in general, or that you don't like discussing any personal things in the workplace.

THE MAILMAN

There are many people in your community whom you know in a peripheral sense. You may see your mailman a few times a week, exchange pleasantries with the local dry cleaner, or have an occasional conversation with the person who works at the corner market. There is no reason why you should feel obligated to tell anyone about your child's sexuality—especially those with whom you have a more surface relationship. At the same time, if you find that a conversation prompts a response indicating that your child is gay, you might decide to answer honestly. You will find that these exchanges, and your decision on how to handle them, will vary. Sometimes being straightforward will come easily, while other times it will just seem easier to gloss over the truth and continue on your way. Your child has these same experiences in their everyday life, and it is absolutely okay for you to trust your gut within each individual experience.

Remember that you are navigating new territory, and you should never feel pressured or obligated to speak to people about anything that you do not want to share. You might make a decision to keep things to yourself in certain situations, yet begin to feel more comfortable down the line. No one should ever judge you for taking time to process this new information. Try not to overthink it, and have patience with yourself. When you do open up to others about your child, remember that it doesn't have to be a huge and serious discussion; their response is informed by your delivery. You will have awkward moments—we all do. Many things will get easier with time and practice, and even the most awkward exchanges will soften with time.

"Once one person knew, everyone knew."

You know how, sometimes when you tell one person, you may as well have told the whole world? Well, that sort of happened to me when I came out. I was seventeen, and a high school senior in a relatively small town in North Carolina. My dad is a rabbi in the Conservative Reconstructionist movement and my mom is an English professor. I should also add that my mom even taught, prior to me coming out, courses like Women and Literature and Gay and Lesbian Literature. Both of my parents, overall, were pretty accepting.

At first, I didn't want others to know, unless I felt ready or had control of the situation. I probably should have known that wasn't going to happen, since my mom told my dad within hours of me coming out to her. It was only a matter of time until others were told. Soon after I came out to my parents, they told a few of their closest friends. One person they told was Deborah, who was well connected to my dad's synagogue. Prior to my coming out, she was a close family friend and involved in life happenings, from Passover seders to hurricanes. In some ways, she was a mother figure to my parents. She had provided our family with wisdom and support in times of need, and it was without question or surprise that my parents would tell her early on.

Once one person in the congregation knew about my sexual orientation, pretty much everyone knew. That's the basis of how our culture works to some degree: You tell one person and they tell a group of people and then another person and so on. When I go back to my parents' home now, regardless of whether I know the person or not, I am pretty sure they have heard about my affinity for men at some level.

The way that others found out forced me to quickly become at peace with my own sexuality, prompting me to let go of control and care less what others thought about me being gay. Truthfully, I have become much more comfortable with others knowing, and feel that my parents sharing the news with our congregation helped bring awareness about the idea of being gay and Jewish to a small, conservative city. It may also have helped others who are thinking about coming out.

When I go home for the popular rosemary potatoes on Thanksgiving or the crispy potato latkes on Hanukkah (and to see my family, of course), I do occasionally attend services. Most of the congregants are aware of me being gay after all these years, but, every once in a while, I do get a lady trying to set me up with a nice Jewish girl. Perhaps they simply missed the memo.

Dan, 29

Q: My child doesn't want to come out to my spouse. What do I do?

A: There are many reasons why your kid may have come out to you, but not to your spouse or your significant other. The most common reasons are that they either feel more comfortable talking with you about personal matters, or that they are worried your partner won't be accepting. The first step in navigating this delicate situation is to talk to your kid about their decision, and ask them if they have a plan. They may want you to be the one to have the initial conversation with your partner, or they may want to wait until they feel confident enough to do it themselves. Make a plan with your child that takes their feelings and needs into consideration, but that also respects the trusting relationship you have with your partner.

If the main issue is that your child is less comfortable speaking to your spouse, they may have asked you to tell your partner on their behalf. This doesn't mean they will never have a larger dialogue with your partner. Uttering those first words to someone is often the hardest moment of coming out, so your child is just looking to you to help them get through that initial step. Explain to your child that you will tell your significant other, but that you are also going to encourage them to speak directly to each other after the fact. When you speak with your partner about what your child has communicated to you, and that they asked you to deliver the news, make sure you express how difficult that initial coming-out moment is for a person. Your partner should know that your child's decision to tell you first isn't a reflection on them as a parent, and the best thing they can do is to express their support for their child. It can be as simple as your partner walking over to your kid, placing a hand on their shoulder, and saying, "I want you to know I love you, no matter what. If you need anything, you say the word." Depending on the relationship that your significant other and your child have, it might be something subtler than that, and that is okay. So long as your partner has voiced or shown support, and your child feels that support, you have all done an incredible job.

If your child has asked you *not* to share the information, there needs to be a larger dialogue that addresses your position within this situation. Trust and patience is extremely important in the moments following coming out, so if your kid is asking you to give them a few weeks to work up the courage, it is best to hold off and respect their wishes. If, however, your child says that they have no intentions of ever telling your significant other, this puts you in a difficult position. If you know that your partner will be supportive of your child and their sexuality, then you should explain to your child that you cannot withhold information from someone with whom you share your life. You can, and should, tell your child that you understand their hesitancy and are willing to give them some time, or help them figure out the best way to approach the conversation, but there has to be a plan for you to feel comfortable as a part of a larger family unit.

If your kid has kept this a secret because your significant other is, in fact, unsupportive, things become a bit more difficult. If this is the case, you should be honest with your child about your concerns. You don't have to pretend that your partner will be accepting if you are fairly certain that they may have a harder time with the information. Talk to your kid and tell them that you will do everything in your power to make the situation as easy as possible. In those first moments, let them know you will stand by their side and help them as they navigate their feelings. A loving and safe environment is crucial in those first stages of coming out, so keeping this between you and your child for a short time may be the best decision. When the time comes that they are ready to have that conversation (or have you initiate that conversation), the main thing to keep consistent is your support of your child. Allow your significant other the room to feel the many feelings that may come along with this information. Remember that their initial reaction is not always indicative of how things will be forever. This is a very hard place to be in, but as much as you can, return to your child with support, and let your significant other know that you are also there to listen, to dialogue, and to figure out the best path forward for everyone involved. Talk to your partner about your family as a whole, and ensure that they know this isn't parent versus child.

Mediating between your child and your significant other, however, should not be a permanent solution. It is fine for you to help both of them as much as you are capable, but we all have our limits. While you are in this mediating space, make sure you have someone else to speak with about your situation. Whether it involves attending PFLAG meetings or simply relying on your best friend or a close family member, you should not have to go through this alone. After a time, this will have to be something that is between your child and your partner. You can still show your support for your child and remain as patient as possible with your significant other, but you need to also remember to take care of yourself.

Q: What will people think?

I remember one day when, on a run to the post office, I wore a T-shirt that said the name of my organization, Everyone Is Gay. Now, I don't generally wear rainbows or blast my gayness all over the place, but I had just gotten the shirt in the mail, and I was so excited that I didn't think about it at all before heading on my way. Since everyone is already in a bad mood at the post office, I was convinced I would be scoffed at, whispered about, and made to feel uncomfortable. However, as is often the case in life, I was pleasantly surprised. When I walked up to the counter, the woman behind the desk screamed (literally, she screamed), "Everyone is gay? That's true! I'm gay! I'm married to a man but what I am saying is that I love rainbows and I love gay people!" We began talking, she asked me more about my organization, and I wound up bringing her a T-shirt of her own a few weeks later! Up until that moment, I had really forgotten that people often surprise you.

—*Dannielle*

A: The truth is, you can never know what another person might think of your kid's sexuality until you are smack in the middle of telling them. Feeling a bit uneasy about some of those first conversations is completely normal; as the parent of a gay child, you, also, will have the experience of coming out. This can be an incredibly helpful experience when it comes to relating to your child, because a lot of your initial worries are exactly what they are feeling when they come out to people in their life. We often think that we have to be very serious in communicating our child's sexuality to others, but that isn't always the case. While you can't control or dictate what another person will think of your child's sexuality, you can approach these discussions with a certain amount of levity. Communicate with others based on the way you are feeling. If you feel confused and you express that you need someone to listen and advise, the person you are speaking to will likely pick up on those needs. If you sit them down and give them a somber speech, they will assume their reaction should also be somber. Don't feel that the conversation needs to happen in a particular way, or at a particular moment; you can talk to your best friend while he is cooking spaghetti and meatballs on a Wednesday evening if that is when the moment feels right! The fact of the matter is, different people will come to this information in varying ways, but when you leave it open for their honest response and questions, you will allow them, in turn, to feel at ease.

Some people will respond perfectly without missing a beat. They will ask questions that make sense to you, they will share stories about their own children, and they will let you know they are there to talk if you need them. Catalina, whose son Daniel came out at age fifteen, received very supportive responses from friends who had previously held less-than-positive views of the gay community. Many of them had known Daniel since he was little, and Catalina felt that, for them, Daniel had given a face to the word *gay*. She said, "It has changed many of our friends, and it has helped them. A lot of them are now very protective of Daniel." Seeing responses like these from friends can be extremely encouraging and will let you know, immediately, that you and your child have support and understanding.

Others will not walk such a perfectly paved path of support right away, and may make comments or ask questions that offend you. Answer their questions as best as you can, and try not to feel pressured or defensive. It is easy to feel angry when someone asks, "Well, how does Matthew even know that he's gay?" Those questions may make you want to shout, "It doesn't matter how he knows! I love him and that is all that matters!" In these moments, remind yourself that you had some of these same questions (the very questions in this book!), and that this is a process for *everyone*, not just your child, and not just yourself. Give these people a fighting chance; don't immediately shut down and stop the conversation. Explain to them that certain things may sound hurtful to you. Talk about your own journey to support your child. Have patience. Many of these not-so-perfect reactions are beginning steps on a path that ends with understanding and unwavering support.

You will, occasionally, have discussions with people who fundamentally disagree with you or your child's life. In these cases, it's best to agree to disagree. It may not be ideal, but so long as they aren't pushing you or your child to believe or behave in a particular way, it is still possible to foster love and respect within such relationships. If, however, you find that someone is pressing you to align your beliefs with their own, that is a greater challenge and may present a barrier in continuing your relationship. Don't expect that response from everyone, though—the majority of people have room in their hearts for a dialogue about differing beliefs. If it does come to a point where you are feeling hurt, remind yourself that you want supportive and loving individuals in your life. Many of your conversations will end up surprising you in very positive ways, and many will teach you wonderful things about people you have known and loved for years.

In the end, this is about your relationship with your child. Work to surround yourself with people who will give you *and* your child the love and support that you both need.

THE BOTTOM LINE

* You are also going to have a coming-out experience when you tell others about your kid's sexuality. This can help you relate to how your kid feels when they come out to others.

* Talk to your child about if (and how) they would like you to communicate their sexuality to others.

* You can support your kid and simultaneously work to remain patient with an unsupportive spouse, but remember to also take care of yourself.

* Others, including friends and family members, will also experience this as a process. Give some room for less-than-perfect first responses, and be willing to answer their questions and talk about their concerns.

* Try as best you can to surround yourself with a community of people who support you *and* your child.

CHAPTER 4: Thinking About the Future

Regardless of your kid's sexuality, you may worry about what their future holds, how you can help them achieve their fullest potential, and how their life will unfold over the next several years. After your kid comes out, however, those questions can sometimes seem unmanageable, unclear, and overwhelming. You may be worried about discrimination, career options, family possibilities, or other questions for which you do not readily have the answers. As a parent, worrying about your children's future is in the job description; feeling out to sea when you are a parent to a gay child is more than understandable. Many of your concerns are brand new, and you may not feel as prepared to handle them.

Luckily for you, your child, and the rest of us, our world is growing and changing for the better, and the amount of support available to answer your questions is larger than it has ever been. It is incredibly important when navigating these concerns to educate yourself and speak to your child about their own vision of their future. Looking outward for support is also endlessly helpful. None of those actions will give you control over the future or a complete and accurate picture of what is to come, but they will allow you to feel less isolated and confused. Your child will ultimately walk their own path in life, but they will do so alongside the support, love, and guidance that you provide. Focus on keeping communication open and gathering information that will help you form a clearer picture of how that future might look. This will help ease some of your concerns and also allow you to look openly and excitedly toward the future together with your child.

Q: I never pictured my child's life to be like this.

I have so many memories of my mother shaking her head at me and saying things like, "But . . . you're so pretty" or "What about your future?" I never understood these comments. Couldn't I be gay and be pretty? And happy? And have a good future? I realized, though, that while I was growing up, she had formed a picture of my future in her head. It was extremely hard for her to shake that picture. She had imagined a very specific future for me for almost twenty years, yet this one thing about me—that I was gay—had changed that picture completely. The fact that

I liked girls made it impossible for her to understand the picture she had created. My mom struggled because she didn't know what my future was anymore.

—Dannielle

A: It is a rare thing for any of us to have one crystal-clear vision of who we will be when we grow up, and for that vision to not only remain constant over our lifetime, but for it to also be the exact way in which our life unfolds. Life doesn't often follow rulebooks, guidelines, or expectations. Frequently, we find ourselves in a particular place in life and we think, "Well, I never could have imagined this, but here I am—and now I couldn't really imagine it any other way." Many times, after we have adjusted to this new reality, we also get a sense that it has always been this way or that it was meant to be this way from the start.

The trickiest part of these dips and curves is in the initial introduction of something new, something unexpected, or something unimagined. Michele, whose daughter Zoe came out at age eighteen, had seen her daughter in many relationships with boys throughout her high school years, so she had formed a clear picture of what Zoe's future might look like. "I could see her being a great mom and having a great husband, lots of kids, a dog," she explained. "I felt like I knew what the next step would be, but then a different picture showed up." You, too, have likely imagined what your child's life would look like as they grew into adulthood. Certainly, those pictures were informed by the things around you, and also by experiences that you have had in your own life. Perhaps some of those pictures also aligned with things that you wished you had been able to achieve when you were their age. You might have imagined them studying a particular subject, wearing a certain style of clothing, getting married, having a family, or having a successful career. If you aren't gay, you likely didn't imagine your child to be gay. If you don't know many gay people in general, you weren't working with the tools to incorporate those possibilities into your thoughts. We think around the things we know. The more knowledge you gather around what a "gay" future might look like, the more you will be able to calm those feelings of confusion.

Ask yourself what, in particular, is throwing that picture of your child's future into disarray. What is it that you are thinking about that makes you feel disoriented? Is it simply the thought of them bringing someone home who is not the gender you had initially expected they would be, or are you connecting their sexual orientation to a whole web of other ideas as they relate to family, behavior, dress, politics, and religion? Break apart the pieces so you can look at them one by one, as opposed to wrestling with a whole pile of tangled feelings. If you find that your biggest hurdle is the overall idea of your son bringing a boy home or your daughter crushing on other girls, recognize that it is okay for your initial response to be fearful, confused, or uncertain. You are not going to feel every perfect, supportive emotion right at the start. Be patient with those initial feelings and fears. Gather the tools you need to adjust to a new (and ever-changing) picture of your child's future.

You need to know more about what this all means, what it might look like, and how it might feel in order to become more at ease in these new surroundings.

There are a lot of different ways that you can begin to better understand new family structures and other life experiences that overlap with the LGBTQ community. Reading books, watching documentaries, and speaking with others who have gone through similar experiences are all excellent ways of engaging with and reflecting on your feelings. Participating more in these activities will help you better navigate this process and start to form that new, and perhaps more flexible, picture of your kid's life. There is a list of suggested videos, books, and other material in the Resources on page 222 that will be of help. Take things one step at a time, because if you have been operating under one set of expectations for the past ten or more years, those new imaginings will not be able to simply snap into place overnight.

If you are connecting your child's sexuality with a multitude of other pieces in the your-kid's-future-identity puzzle, hold on a moment. There is nothing about your kid's sexuality that necessarily informs the other elements that make them who they are. While sexuality informs family structure or career path for some, that is not always the case. When it comes to the overall layout of their future, your child's desires would be certain to surprise you even if they weren't gay! The best thing you can do when it comes to these larger questions is try to talk to your kid. Instead of assuming that their sexuality is determinant of their interests in religion or politics or family in any particular way, ask them! Ask them what their thoughts are on family or career, see what inspires them, and use their responses to help inform and reshape your imagining of their future. Remember that what motivates us in one chapter of our lives may be very different from what motivates us in another. Try to digest your child's reality as something that exists right now, in this moment. The hopes and dreams that we have for ourselves change over the years, so we must be willing to accept changes in those hopes, dreams, and desires for the ones we love, and be patient with ourselves as we make those adjustments.

Q: Will my child be interested in different things now?

A: For a lot of people, coming out isn't only about sexuality; it's also about beginning to understand the larger picture of who they are through a new lens. This doesn't always result in a severe shift in interests, and some people will come out and retain all of their previous hobbies, styles, and preferences. Others, though, may find that once they are more confident in expressing their sexuality, they may also begin to recognize other areas in their life in which they weren't quite being themselves. Your child may explore new ways of dressing, read different books, listen to different music, or begin hanging out with some new people. This process of self-discovery is very personal and is different for everyone. Don't assume that, just because of their sexuality, your kid will suddenly want to join the theater department instead of playing basketball, or will now need a supply of black T-shirts.

If you are feeling overwhelmed by the fact that your kid has decided to cut her hair short or isn't watching his favorite television show anymore, that is okay—and very understandable. You have always known certain things about your kid, and are now feeling unsure of where these changes are coming from and why you were unable to anticipate them. Depending on the journey that your child is on, things can sometimes feel very drastic and out of line with past behavior. In those instances, it is important to take a step back so that you can view the larger trajectory of your child's life and see this exploration as a part of the larger whole. Some of these new interests will flourish and others will come and go as they get a firmer grasp on what makes them who they are. Robbie, who came out to his family when he was fifteen, said that he initially viewed the coming-out experience as the "Big Turning Point," and thought it was very important to reevaluate everything in his life in this new light. After a while, though, he said that he kept finding himself going back to things that had been a big part of his life before coming out. "Coming out didn't change who I was as a person," he reflected, "and the things I was interested in before coming out resurfaced."

We have said this many times already, but it always bears repeating: Ask questions. If you are noticing new patterns or behaviors and you want to better understand them, you can (and should) talk to your child. Try not to ask them in a way that implies you are unhappy with the changes or in a manner that suggests you don't believe this is the "real" them. Instead, ask open-ended questions like, "So, where did you meet Todd and Jennifer? They seem really nice," or "I have been noticing you are over the old Adidas sneakers and really loving Converse—are they more comfortable or do you just like the way they look?" Engaging them in conversations like these helps you better understand their reasoning, and helps them feel supported.

Also, let them lead with specifics. Instead of saying, "Do you want to go to that store where all the employees have nose rings and pink hair?" say, "Do you want to go shopping? Where would you like to go?" No one ever wants to feel that part of their identity is shaping the opinions others have of them. Even if your child did want to shop at that store with the pink-haired, pierced employees, your assumption that this is where they want to go might make them feel robbed of their ability to assert their independence and make their own choices, and may also make them feel that you are judging them based on their sexuality. Leave them the space to surprise you.

Finally, allow yourself a learning curve. You are going to have experiences in which you buy them something they might have loved three months ago, but now isn't "them" at all. This isn't a reflection on you, and doesn't mean you don't know your kid—it simply means that they are working toward understanding their identity and may not be aware of how that shift is impacting you. In those moments when you feel unsure, scared, or lost, think about the parts of your child that you know will never change: their passion, their values, that silly grin that they get despite themselves when they are playfully embarrassed, the way they click their pen while they do their homework, the jokes they tell their little cousin, and how much they love you. Find those constants and hold on to them to help steady yourself at a time when other things are changing. This is all a part of growing up and, though some of it may hinge on sexuality, a lot of it is just about your child discovering the world around them.

Q: My child is bisexual. Does this mean they can later choose to be straight?

A: If your child has come out to you as bisexual, this likely means that they are expressing an attraction to more than one gender. That attraction may be physical, emotional, romantic, or any combination therein. If what you are asking is, "If my son just said he likes boys and girls, does that mean he might end up with a girl?" then the answer is, it's definitely possible! However, even if your son winds up getting married to a woman, there is a good chance he will still identify as bisexual. Partnering with someone whose gender is different from your own does not mean that you are "straight"; it means that you are committing to that person and that person's gender at this point in your life. If you have been with

"How I see my future"

When I first came out to my parents in a letter from college, they called me to talk. They said that they would love and support me no matter what, and I felt a huge wave of relief. My sexual orientation wasn't something we talked about until almost a year later, but the wall had been breached after many years of attempting to hide important parts of my life from them.

A few days after our phone call, I received a letter from my mother. When I saw the return address, I was worried—would they have changed their minds about being able to accept me? Would they not be sure they wanted my girlfriend to visit, or feel worried about conflicts with their strong religious beliefs?

However, as soon as I saw my mother's cursive writing on both sides of a piece of notebook paper, I knew that my decision to come out to them had been the right one. My mother wrote, again, that my parents loved me no matter what, and that she wanted me to have it in writing for when times were tough. On the second page, she asked a question that had come to her mind since our call: How would my sexuality affect my future plans?

At first, I was taken aback by this question—I had known I was gay for about six years, and had already gone through the "major life decisions" phase that follows high school with that information in mind. I went to a college far from home not only because I felt that the school was right for me, but because the distance gave me the freedom to test out my new identity without the worry of what people I had known my whole life would say. I had based many of my course selections on learning more about sexuality, and had even selected a major research project based on my interest in portrayals of queer characters in literature. I joined the gay-straight alliance at my college and developed a close-knit circle of gay friends.

My orientation *had* affected my future plans—but in the sense that I was enjoying a period of discovery and belongingness that I had never felt growing up in the South. In other ways, deciding to be entirely out was insignificant to how I wanted to live—I still wanted to play sports, pursue a degree in literature, and find someone to spend my life with.

But for my parents, coming out added new information to their ideas of what my life would be like. I wondered if they were waiting for the other shoe to drop—for me to suddenly denounce everything I had valued up to that point. I wasn't planning to; in fact, I caught some resistance about my commitment to Christianity from gay friends. However, being asked about my future plans by my mother did make me think seriously about how much being gay does affect my decisions—for instance, to sometimes walk not holding my partner's hand, or on what jobs to pursue based on state laws and employer benefits that are available to me and my partner. I have also become increasingly interested in serving as an activist.

I didn't have an answer for my mother about my future when I was in college, but I think that my answer has become clearer to her over the years as she has seen my decisions about where to live and work.

My parents have now seen what kind of person I value building my life with, and they see that my partner is the person who takes care of me and supports me. She is now a fixture at family gatherings—my dad shows her how to properly tie the boat to the dock, and my mom employs her as a sous-chef at Thanksgiving with all of her own daughters. Most important, they treat her as they would any of my sisters' spouses. In that sense, my future plans remain completely unchanged: to pursue my career while continuing to build my relationship with my family, and to begin a family of my own.

Kate, 24

more than one person in your life, you will understand that your feelings for your current partner don't mean that you never had any attractions or feelings before that person came into your life. You would never say, "I am only attracted to women who wear glasses" if your wife wears glasses, because there were likely many people with perfect eyesight in whom you were interested in prior to getting married!

If you are asking this question simply because you are confused about bisexuality and what, exactly, it means, be aware that it means different things to different people. Some of us like only one gender, some of us like many genders, and some of us fluctuate in our attractions over the course of our lives. Bisexuality, at its root, implies being attracted to men and women. As we will discuss in more detail in chapter 7, however, there are gender identities that fall outside of "man" and "woman." The term *pansexual*, closely linked with bisexual, describes an individual who is attracted to men, women, and individuals of different gender identities—or those who choose not to identify with any gender at all. It is important to note that liking more than one gender doesn't change based on the person or people we date—bisexuality (and pansexuality), for many, just means that gender isn't an element that determines attraction.

You may have come to this question because you are hoping that your child has a higher chance of pairing with someone of a gender different from their own. The real question to pose to yourself, though, is *why* you are hoping for this in the first place, and how this line of thinking may affect your kid. Perhaps you are worried about their safety, or are having a hard time envisioning their future in this light; maybe you have concerns that align with religious or political beliefs. These are all valid issues and are addressed in further detail in the following chapters. Your concerns, though, should be expressed and discussed with attention to specifics, and not simply delivered in a blanket statement of "I'd rather you were straight," or "If you like boys and girls, why can't you just make this easier on all of us?" Those kinds of statements can be very hurtful.

Just like any other person, your kid does not have control over their feelings or attractions. If they have come out to you as bisexual, this means that they are feeling those attractions toward more than just one gender. That cannot be swept under the rug. When feelings are hidden away from view, they grow stronger and stronger until they reappear. Asking your child to choose, or suggesting that they *should* choose, will likely only result in making them feel guilty, angry, and isolated.

Rather than trying to redirect their attractions in a way that will make *you* feel better, engage with them so that you can better understand what they have communicated with you. If your child enters into a "straight" relationship, do not ask them if that means they are no longer bisexual. Identity is a complicated thing, and making them feel that whom they date erases a part of that identity will make them feel self-conscious and misunderstood. Frame your questions around wanting to better understand your child, rather than asking them questions that you hope will be answered in a particular way. You can say to your son, "I am working really hard to understand this part of you so that I can be the best parent possible. I think that the more I understand, the easier this will be on both of us, and I want you to know that even though this is a process for me, I love you every single step of the way." Those words express your true feelings and confusions but also include the fact that you are both working together and that you share a common goal of wanting to better understand each other.

Q: Will my child always be viewed differently? I worry that they will face discrimination.

My father never had any religious, political, or moral issues with my sexuality. He did, however, talk to me about wanting me to be happy, and his fear that I would perhaps walk a harder path. When we first had that conversation, I was only seventeen and I didn't understand how discrimination would ever impact me, personally. I had surrounded myself with open-minded friends and planned to move to New York City, where, in my mind, this discrimination simply didn't occur. As you might imagine, I was wrong. Holding my girlfriend's hand would generally cause extended stares from passersby, I was catcalled more than once for kissing a girl in public, and I slowly became aware of the fact that, in a lot of places, I wouldn't be afforded certain basic human rights such as the right to marry. Those experiences taught (and continue to teach) me two things. First, that my dad was right: when something sets you apart from what others expect, things can be harder. Second, that those experiences were shaping me in ways I could have never imagined. Yes,

I was upset by certain occurrences, and I still feel frustrated in moments when I know that I am being viewed as "different." However, those experiences also brought to light things that made me question the world around me in very useful ways; I learned to challenge ideas and stereotypes and to get to know other people on much deeper, more nuanced levels. I feel like, though the path may be more difficult in certain ways, it is also much more enlightening.

—*Kristin*

A: When it comes to being viewed as "different," our brains tend to focus on the negative. You don't want your child to feel that they are less important, less valued, or less *anything* than another person because of the way that others may treat them. You want to ensure that your kid has equal access to anything and everything they might seek, regardless of sexuality. We would love to be able to tell you not to worry, and that your child will be able to navigate the ins and outs of growing up gay without ever having to feel like an outsider, without ever having to fight for basic human rights, and without ever having to worry about speaking openly and honestly about their identity. However, those statements are likely untrue. As a planet, we are on a positive trajectory toward change that will allow your child to live in a more equal world than was once possible. Within a general population, though, there will always be others who treat us differently based on many factors. Most of us grow up in very monochromatic environments, and we are led to expect the rest of the world will look just the same.

You have likely had at least one experience that caused others to view you as "different," regardless of your sexuality; many of us have these experiences in some form on a regular basis. If you are a woman, you will likely recall moments throughout your life when others (generally with nothing but good intentions!) offered to carry a heavy box for you or "helped" you parallel park. This is only one example of how our identities inform the opinions of others. It is possible that your kid has already faced some form of discrimination in their lifetime, even if it wasn't directly applicable to being gay. As a parent, you want your children to be safe from hatred, and you also want them to live in a world where they will have equal rights. These are valid concerns.

Some of your worries won't immediately resonate with your child. It can be exceptionally hard for them to imagine how tax or adoption laws will affect them when they are figuring out how to navigate the prom and study for a history exam. It won't be helpful to barrage your child with a long list of items that you are thinking about when it comes to their future, or to attempt to get their concerns aligned with your own. Begin by addressing these concerns for yourself. Simply shrugging off your worries as something that you will deal with "later" or "when the time comes" doesn't often work—and can lead to a lot of sleepless nights where you toss and turn thinking about the possibilities that lie ahead.

Try to look at your concerns regarding discrimination in two lights: social and legal. Social discrimination refers to those moments when your child is stared at or made to feel different or inadequate in public settings. This is the kind of discrimination that targets them emotionally or physically—that might put them in danger or make them feel they have to hide a part of themselves to remain safe or not judged. Legal discrimination refers to instances when they might be denied a job, housing, or other basic human rights because of their sexuality.

With regard to social discrimination, having general conversations with your child about their experience is a great way to gauge how they are feeling and what they have faced in their own community. Those topics make a great bridge toward explaining that you sometimes worry that they will have a harder life, and that these worries are occasionally hard for you to manage. They should know that you have feelings surrounding their happiness and safety, and even if they aren't able to understand them all at this point in time, they will understand that you support them and want them to be happy. Rather than telling them to be "safe," suggest that they remain aware of the environment around them. Ask them when they feel safest and which places make them uncomfortable. Talk to them about how you might have handled a situation in which someone said something hurtful, or when your behavior or appearance resulted in long stares from others. There is no "right" way to respond to these moments, but talking about the possibilities will help your child feel more equipped if they are faced with those situations. The thing that is most important when it comes to experiencing hurtful words or stares is having strength and peace within ourselves. The more confident and secure your child is able to feel with their own identity, the easier it becomes for them to handle these situations. Encourage them to talk to you, and make sure that they know you are always willing to listen and to help in any way you can if they are feeling unsafe or judged in the larger community.

When it comes to legal discrimination, knowledge is power. LGBTQ rights are changing at a pace that is often hard to keep up with, but there are newsfeeds, social media outlets, and other resources that exist solely to keep people up to date on the ever-changing landscape. Look into the laws in your own state. Anti-discrimination policies are crucial in protecting our rights, and looking at the policies at your own place of employment is a great way to start learning about these intricacies. It is not enough for a school or workplace policy to issue protection from general discrimination. Using specific and inclusive language in the policies is vital. These policies should include words such as *sexuality*, *gender*, *religion*, *race*, *gender identity*, and *disability*. We have devoted an entire section of our Resources on page 229 to combating legal discrimination and helping you remain informed on the changing laws in our world. Use these resources to inform yourself, and share specific facts with your kid as you begin to learn more about the LGBTQ legal landscape. Even if your child doesn't take in all of the information, knowing some details about what is happening in the world around them will often spark their interest in learning more, and their knowledge on these issues is key in helping them as they grow up.

"I wanted her to know there wasn't anything wrong with her."

My daughter, Parisa, is an only child. Having her was a profound experience for me, and I've always been extremely close to her. When Parisa was very young, even four or five, she self-identified as a boy. I knew that there was something different, but I didn't worry. She was just my little girl, and we did the same things we always had. As she got older, Parisa did not like to dress in girls' clothes. I don't know if I'd call her a tomboy necessarily, because she liked to do little girl things, too, but there was some indication that she wasn't completely comfortable with identifying as a girl or a woman. So I just waited. I just treated her like my child. There was no difference day to day.

I grew up in rural Maryland in an era when, if you were gay, you were beat up at school. There was a lot of discrimination and prejudice. I had a lot of gay friends growing up, and it's something they hid. If it was revealed, they were harassed and physically abused at school. Northern California, where we live, is much more gay-friendly than just about any other place in the country, and so my immediate concerns for her being harassed or abused weren't quite as strong. My main concern was that she didn't think that there was something wrong with her, and so my sort of indirect message to her was that nobody had the right to define her. You can be exactly who you want—that was the refrain. I didn't want to say, "Oh, do you think you might be gay?" because I didn't know. I had no way of placing this in the spectrum of what was going to happen, so I just wanted to make sure that whatever happened, she was comfortable with who she was.

After she got on social networks, she announced one day on Facebook to all her contacts that she was gay. She didn't tell me. I went to her to say, "Hey, I read your Facebook today." And she said, "Well, I figured you sort of knew, so it wasn't a big deal." It was something that she needed to express, and she did. Since then, it's just not been an issue; at the end of the day, she's still my daughter. She's still Parisa, and nothing's changed.

People have asked me, "Would you prefer if she was straight?" It's a funny question, because my personal preference is that I just want her to be her—I have never had any issue with her sexuality. I do know from my own experience, though, that in the rest of the United States and the world, being gay is not always accepted. I made it clear to her that she's been very fortunate to grow up in an area where there is so much acceptance, but that it's not like that everywhere and that she's going to have to be careful. If she moves somewhere else, she's going to have to understand the landscape.

The thing about Parisa is that she's seventeen going on thirty. She's very mature, self-reliant, confident, and aware—much more so than I ever was at that age—and I think she gets it. Parisa's success in life has always been determined through connecting with people and forming relationships and support groups. Her gayness is subordinate to her ability to connect with people, straight and gay. I don't think being gay defines her, and I don't see her as gay so much as just Parisa. She's a very nice, lovable person, and that defines her. She just happens to be gay.

Chris, 48

Q: I'm worried that my child won't ever have a family.

A: When we first come out, many of us aren't in a place where we know if we would like to get married or have children. Even if we are, those desires and wants and imaginings often shift throughout the course of our lives. If you start to worry about your child's sexuality and how it might impact their future family structure, there are three things to focus on: first, what we mean when we say "family"; second, how our wants might not overlap in the exact same patterns as the wants and needs of those we love; and third, how the logistical and legal landscape may affect certain family structures.

Family doesn't have to mean having a different-gendered partner, 2.5 kids, and a really adorable dog named Pickles. That sounds like an awesome family (especially Pickles), but it is just one definition of a word that can mean many things to many people. Family, simply put, is created by people who love one another. Single parents and their children, grandparents who raise grandchildren, foster families, groups of tight-knit friends who support each other through the ups and downs of life—all of these structures create families.

Your child may not want to have the same exact family structure that you have chosen, and they might have a different idea of what family means. That idea might stay with them forever, or it might shift depending on the people who come into their life over time. The best possible thing you can do when you are worrying about these differences is to open the lines of communication with your kid without putting pressure on them to align with your wants, or to "know" exactly what they want for the rest of their life. Talk to them. Ask questions. Make sure they know that your number-one concern is their happiness, and not expecting them to fit a preexisting mold of what you had envisioned for their future. Do not present your idea of family as the only option, and be careful to make sure that they know that many possibilities for having a family are open to them regardless of their sexuality.

If your child wants to marry or have children one day, there are a lot of choices available to them. Same-sex marriage laws are being passed with increasing frequency, as are adoption laws. Many couples choose to get married in places where gay marriage is legal, or have commitment ceremonies in places whose laws don't yet recognize their union. These couples sometimes choose to adopt children, use a surrogate to carry a biological child if neither is able to carry, or have children through sperm donors if one partner is able to carry a child. The option of committing to a partner or having a family is not ruled out for your kid just because they are gay.

If you keep your focus on loving and supporting your child, it will allow them to feel more comfortable talking to you about their future vision of family. Those conversations will give you the opportunity to better understand them, to help them make important decisions, and to remain an integral part of their life. When you say you want your child to have a family, generally what you are saying is that you want for them to find happiness. Happiness, though, finds us in many different ways. Work toward a place where you can accept that your child may find happiness in ways you never dreamed for them, but that with your love and support, they will be able to understand themselves and their path to happiness much more clearly.

THE BOTTOM LINE

* Talk to your child about their future as much as they will allow. Don't assume that anything will be foreclosed to them because of their sexuality.

* Work to understand that our visions of our future shift and change as we grow, and are generally not constant or predictable.

* Ask your child about ways in which they may have encountered discrimination. Understanding their day-to-day experiences will be helpful in navigating a larger landscape.

* Family means many things to many people. Your kid may have a family that looks different from your own in many ways, but that doesn't mean they won't find their own happiness.

* Ensure that your kid knows that your top priority is their happiness, and not for them to fit the exact vision you had for their future.

CHAPTER 5: The Birds and the Bees

Some parents feel very comfortable talking to their children about sex. Many, however, are hesitant when it comes to having any discussion about sexual matters, and they, like their kids, dread these conversations. Whether you are on the comfortable or mortified end of the sex-talk spectrum, you are now faced with the prospect of engaging in a dialogue about kinds of sex with which you may have little to no experience. This can be a daunting task, as we are often intimidated by what we do not know.

This chapter will help alleviate some of the more common misperceptions about people in the gay community when it comes to sex, and also give you the tools to feel more at ease in talking about *all* kinds of sex with your children. The more you know, the more open you can be with your child. The more open you are able to be with your child about sex, the easier it will be for them to talk to you about their questions and concerns. Many teens say that their parents were their biggest influence when it came to making decisions about sex. What you say *does* matter—and what you leave unsaid can sometimes matter even more.

———

Q: Does being gay mean my child is going to be promiscuous?

A: Simply put: no. Your child's sexuality does not inform how often they engage (or want to engage) in sex, nor does it inform the emotions that they attach to having sex. There are a wide variety of sexual behaviors and interests within the "straight" community, and it is the same for those of varying sexualities. People are people, and our desires do not hinge on only one facet of our identity.

It is also important to recognize that promiscuity doesn't automatically align with something negative. Having "casual sex" may mean a lot of different things to you, depending on who you are. There are people who view casual sex as risky, irresponsible, and immoral, and others who are comfortable remaining uncommitted and having sex with multiple partners, while also making safe, informed decisions. Your views on having sex may not align with your child's at this point in time, but the only way you will be able to know about their views is by talking to them, openly, about their feelings.

When you have that conversation with your child, avoid overlaying judgment or assumptions in your words or your tone. Take some time before you approach the subject to think about your own views of sex. When and how did they originate? Have you always felt the same about sex and emotional attachment? Are your views rooted in moral or religious beliefs, or are you just concerned about safety? When you talk to your child, you might say something like, "You are at a point in your life when you may be thinking about having sex. I know it isn't something that we talk about a lot, but at the end of the day, it is important that we both understand each other and communicate about these things because they are very important." Tell your child how *you* feel about sex, and be honest.

Gibson, who is seventeen, said that the door was always open for him to talk to his parents about sex. "I never felt like it was dirty or something that I couldn't talk about," he said. "I felt like it was something that was great and that I was free to do as long as I was protecting myself." Your opinions on sex may be a bit different from Gibson's parents, but that doesn't mean you can't be open to discussion. Talk through the questions that you asked yourself before you begin speaking with your kid; reflect on your own journey and beliefs. Your honesty on these issues will inspire respect, and that respect will inspire deeper thought, more meaningful dialogue, and an increased sense of responsibility from your child.

Even if they don't tie emotions to sex in the same way that you do, your child will value and consider your perspective. Plus, any discussion surrounding sex is an additional opportunity for you to educate them on safe-sex practices.

Your concerns about your child's sexual behavior should not, and need not, be directed only toward their sexuality. When it comes to safe-sex practices, being specific and inclusive of all sexual activity is important (refer to the next question on safe sex to learn more about this). Your child is at an age—or will soon be at an age—when sex comes up in conversation and in experimentation, so it's important to help them consider what sex means to them. Be open to what they have to say, and remember that their sexuality does not determine their interest in sex or their choices surrounding it. At the end of the day, their body is their body, and the best thing you can provide them with is honest dialogue about your own experience and tools to make safe, informed decisions.

Q: **How do I talk to my child about safe sex?**

I never learned how to have safe sex. I am sure that I had a few health classes that talked about condoms and rattled off a lot of facts about scary diseases I might get if I did the wrong thing with the wrong person—but no one ever mentioned what to do if I wasn't having sex with a boy. I didn't know if I was supposed to protect myself and, if I was, I had never heard of any ways in which I could do so. My parents didn't know that I was gay until after I was sexually active, and I don't think they ever even considered talking to me about having safe "gay" sex. My mom didn't want me to be gay in the first place, so she certainly wasn't going to be a source of information. I was lucky enough to get through those before-I-knew years unscathed, but I would have definitely made different, more informed decisions had I known anything about protecting myself.

—Kristin

A: Many parents are nervous about talking to their children about *any* kind of sex and also operate under the misconception that by avoiding the topic entirely, their child will simply not have sex with anyone. Kids have sex. Even when forbidden from doing so, kids have sex. When given the tools to understand sex, what it means, how it works, and how to practice it responsibly, they are much safer and more prepared to make important decisions than they would be if they were operating blindly.

The majority of middle and high schools are not equipped to handle the logistics or the precautions that are necessary for your child to become and remain informed and safe—especially when it comes to sex that isn't heterosexual. What's more, many teens name their parents as their resource for information on practicing safe sex. You are wise to inform yourself so *you* can be the one who discusses these issues with your kid. What you say, and how you say it, is endlessly important.

The way you approach talking about safe sex will depend entirely on your own comfort level and your relationship with your kid. If talking about sex comes easily to you, then your child may also be comfortable discussing such topics—in which case, you can skip on ahead to Safe Sex 101 on page 122 and chat away! Perhaps, though, despite your own ease discussing sexual activity, your child is uncomfortable—or maybe you are both a little uneasy around the topic. If this is the case, it is entirely reasonable to rely on the old adage, "Know your audience."

Oluremi, who is eighteen and out to both of her parents, said her mother took a different route than most when approaching safe sex. "Luckily, my mom understood that I wasn't really one for talking, but knew I would read anything put in front of me," she said. Oluremi's mom communicated most of her thoughts on safe sex with her daughter through e-mail, which she knew would make the exchange of information easier. The "sex talk" doesn't—and most likely shouldn't—have to be one long conversation held at the dinner table. It can be something that evolves over time, perhaps in a letter or over the course of several smaller discussions. Prepare yourself with the information that you will need, and communicate in the way that you think will bring the highest level of comfort to both you and your child.

According to Dr. Justine Shuey, a globally recognized sex expert, the earlier you start talking to your kids, the easier things will be for you later in the game. "The most important thing you

This Is a Book for Parents of Gay Kids

can accomplish is to become an askable parent," she says. This does not mean you have to have all of the answers, or that you need to be comfortable talking to your child about everything (or telling them what *you* do sexually), but that you are approachable and open to questions. If you don't know an answer, research it together. Share reliable, medically and factually accurate sources with your child. Help them find the answers. "When I teach educators, I teach them to first say 'Good question,'" Shuey explains. "That is your moment to think about your answer before you laugh or blurt out something silly or negative." She urges parents to respond positively to their kid's questions so they can continue to be approachable. If you don't know the answer, aren't comfortable, or are unsure if the answer is correct, she suggests saying, "I don't know, but I can find out for you" or "I don't know, but this is where you can find that answer."

Some facts provided by Dr. Shuey are collected into Safe Sex 101 on the following pages. They won't answer every question your child might have, but they will give you an excellent start to understanding more about addressing safe sex that is not just heterosexual.

Q: **Should I be concerned about sexually transmitted infections like AIDS?**

A: You should be concerned about STIs, including HIV and AIDS, just as you would be if your child were not gay. The main cause for elevated concern is the lack of proper safe-sex

SAFE SEX 101

+ Sexually transmitted infections (STIs) are the same as sexually transmitted diseases (STDs). Both terms refer to illnesses that have a significant probability of being transmitted between individuals by means of sexual behavior, including vaginal intercourse, oral sex, and anal sex. The Centers for Disease Control and Prevention (CDC) now uses the term STI instead of STD because *infection* is a less stigmatizing word.

+ All sexual behaviors have some level of risk. Individuals need to know how to manage the risks to make sex safer. STIs do not discriminate. It doesn't matter who is having sex with whom—what matters is what is touching what. Oral sex, anal sex, vaginal sex, sharing sex toys, mutual masturbation, and a wide range of other sexual behaviors all have risks.

+ There is no such thing as "gay sex" or "lesbian sex." People engage in a variety of sexual behaviors, and orientation doesn't necessarily determine what someone might enjoy sexually.

There are four different types of sexually transmitted infections:

bacterial infections—chlamydia, gonorrhea, nongonococcal urethritis, syphilis

viral infections—herpes simplex virus (HSV), human papilloma virus (HPV), viral hepatitis, human immunodeficiency virus (HIV)

protozoal infections— trichomoniasis (trich)

parasitic infections— pubic lice (crabs), scabies

Some STIs, such as genital herpes or HPV, can lead to genital warts or cancers. They are transmitted via skin-to-skin contact, through bodily fluids, through contact with an infected sore, etc. Some infections, such as scabies or pubic lice, can be transmitted simply via close contact. Many people believe oral sex is safe sex, but unless they are taking appropriate precautions, oral sex can transmit gonorrhea, herpes, HPV, and other infections in the throat. Anilingus (oral sex on an anus) can increase the risk of hepatitis and other gastrointestinal infections. Anal sex and vaginal sex can transmit a variety of STIs.

While many infections can be treated, they can't all be cured, particularly viral infections. Even with some bacterial infections, drug resistance is becoming a problem, making treatment more difficult. Moreover, because many sexually transmitted infections (such as HPV and chlamydia) are asymptomatic, people with no signs or symptoms may still transfer a sexually transmitted infection to their partner. However, prevention is easier than treatment, and there are vaccines that protect against some strains of HPV and hepatitis. In addition, males who have sex with other males should also consider getting a meningitis vaccination.

There are many ways to make sex safer:

Male condoms

+ Condoms should be worn over the penis to prevent the exchange of bodily fluids. Male condoms come in latex and non-latex varieties. Latex and non-latex condoms made of polyurethane or polyisoprene protect against pregnancy and sexually transmitted infections. Non-latex condoms made of lambskin, sheepskin, or other animal skins offer protection only against pregnancy but do not offer any protection against sexually transmitted infections.

+ Flavored male condoms can be used during fellatio (oral sex on a penis). Flavored condoms are not meant for penetrative sex of the vagina or anus.

+ Oil-based lubricants can break down latex-based condoms and dental dams, and should be avoided. Most male condoms have silicone lubricant on them. Some are non-lubricated and lubricant can be added.

+ Avoid condoms with spermicides and spermicidal lubricants (particularly those with nonoxynol-9), as they can break down the cell walls in the vagina and anus, making it easier to transmit bacteria and viruses.

+ Use only one condom at a time. Male and female condoms should never be used at the same time. It is important to remember that male condoms do not offer 100 percent protection, and some sexually transmitted infections can be transmitted via skin-to-skin contact.

Female condoms

+ Also known as insertable condoms or internal condoms, female condoms are inserted in the vagina to prevent pregnancy, STIs, and HIV.

+ Female condoms can also be used during receptive anal intercourse. To insert anally, remove the inner ring and insert in the anus, with the outer ring sitting outside the body. To remove, twist the outer ring and pull out.

+ Because female condoms are made of a non-latex material, lubricant can be used.

+ Female condoms do not offer complete protection against all STIs.

Dental dams

+ Dental dams are thin sheets of latex or non-latex material used during cunnilingus (oral sex on a vulva) or anilingus (oral sex on an anus).

+ Some dental dams are flavored. A drop of flavored lubricant can be used on the outside to make it taste better, and a drop of water-based lubricant can be used on the inside to make it feel better.

+ Do not use oil-based lubricants on latex dental dams.

Lubricants

+ Lubricants can be used in safer-sex practices to reduce
  friction, lessening the possibilities of broken condoms
  or skin abrasions.

+ Water-based lubricants are go-to lubricants, safe for use
  on anything (except in eyes or ears). Water-based lubricants
  can be used for oral, anal, and vaginal sex or on sex toys.

+ Silicone lubricant is found on most condoms and while it's
  safe for anal and vaginal sex, it doesn't taste very good for
  oral sex and it might stain sheets and clothing. It is water-
  proof, so it's safe for use in the shower, but should never
  be used on silicone sex toys because it will break down the
  toys when the silicones react with each other.

+ Flavored lubricants are meant for oral sex and should be
  used externally only.

+ Oil-based lubricants can break down latex and irritate the
  vagina; therefore, they should never be used for penetrative
  sex or with condoms or dental dams.

"What my parents taught me about sex"

When I was about ten or twelve, my family made one of our regular journeys up to nearby Montreal, an hour away from our suburban home in upstate New York. Back in those days (the roaring '90s), it was common for American families to pillage Canadian shopping centers with their plentiful greenbacks. If I recall correctly, this particular trip was to procure one of those can't-live-without electric kettles, which, up until then, we seemed to be fine living without.

At some point during our meanderings around the Canadian mall, my father and I split off from my mom and sister and found ourselves passing a magazine kiosk. My father seized this as an opportunity to educate me about the birds and the bees. He reached for a *Playboy* magazine and opened to the centerfold beauty, some blonde type sprawled out across the two pages. I don't remember precisely how she looked, but I do recall my father pointing to her and saying, "In a few years, you're going to go crazy for this. You should know now before the hormones hit."

I was speechless. I can't recall another time when my father was so off the mark.

Today, that moment of father/son bonding seems remote, fuzzy—a rare moment when the topic of sex was brought up deliberately. Even more rare was any talk about homosexuality. There were several occasions when my parents discovered pornography on the computer, but the moments were brief, their reaction curt and temperate, and nothing more was said.

Of the few things said about sex, what was beneficial was my father's emphasis on loving my partner in a sexually active relationship. When my dad talked about sex, he focused on being sensible and safe about it, and that advice was directly translatable. What's more, he never took any issue with gay men. He had even served around gay men in the merchant navy, and would often share stories that cast them in a positive light. I have largely adopted his "live and let live" attitude, which helped me get through those adolescent years, fraught as they were with the self-doubt common to LGBTQ youth.

My relationship with my dad has since matured, and I would say that, by having a gay son, he has learned nearly as much about sexuality (though not sex) as I have. While I never got an ideal parental introduction to sex, I am thankful it wasn't any worse.

Dean, 26

"My first thought was AIDS."

When our son first told me he was gay, one of my first thoughts was AIDS. I know that is largely a generational thing, because I saw too many friends die from AIDS in the '80s and early '90s. Now people are more knowledgeable. But still, that was my first thought. And because he was only sixteen, I worried about predatory older men. How many stereotypes could I conjure up in one worry?

I am of a generation that hasn't given much thought to gay sex. For straight, sheltered people my age (though not me, specifically), I think there is still what we might describe as an "ick" factor. While we may want to feel that sex is both "God's gift to humans," and the most natural of behaviors, I don't know that, as parents, we can easily apply that to our own children. We diapered them, after all. The prospect of anyone, whether age appropriate or not, looking lustfully at your child (of any age) is, at first, horrifying. I realize I find it just as hard to imagine my straight children (late teens to early twenties) having sex. So, better not to try to "envision" them being intimate with anyone, gay or straight. The details are none of our business.

So what to talk about with them? I am sure I don't have the answers, but, when in doubt: condoms. During the many wrenching conversations I had with my son when he first came out, I made him promise me he would always practice safe sex. That means using a condom. He was a little taken aback, at first, that I was serious in wanting him to promise this. His response was, "So you think I'm going to get AIDS, too? Being gay isn't enough of an issue?"

A year or so after this early discussion, I got a panicked call from my husband. He was doing the laundry and found a condom in our son's pocket. In truth, we weren't sure what to do. But I do think we would have felt the same way whether this had been the pants pocket of our gay or straight son. I don't think either of us was ready to know our son was sexually active. Although if he had a condom, perhaps he was more responsible and ready than we thought. Anyway, I got the short stick and was the one to talk with our son. I practiced: "We found this in your laundry. We're glad that you're being responsible, and just want to make sure you're emotionally ready to be sexually active." I sounded just like Dr. Phil. I got up the nerve to go in to talk with him, and got that whole practiced speech out. He looked at me incredulously. "They were giving them away for free at the club, Mom. I haven't used it!" I still have the speech, in case it comes up again.

I'm sure my son will want to talk with me less as he gets older. Obviously, when he's off at college, he will be relying on me less and less for advice. I've never thought I was especially gifted in providing relationship advice, but I do wonder whether his dating men gives us more in common than I initially thought. And as long as he knows that the door is open, literally or figuratively, I plan to be available. But not prying! I'm hoping he'll find someone to love and marry, just as I hope for my straight sons.

Elizabeth, 50

education many LGBTQ youth receive in schools. While hetero-sexual youth are sometimes afforded health education that includes extremely vital safe-sex practices, LGBTQ youth are often overlooked entirely in such lessons. However, since no two health education classes are the same, and some overlook safe-sex practices for *all* individuals, your concern about your child's safety—regardless of their sexuality—is valid. But that doesn't mean your gay kid is in grave danger of contracting an STI; it means you should help educate them so that they can remain safe and protected.

In the late 1970s and early 1980s, the world saw an outbreak of the AIDS virus for the very first time. As it was a new disease, people were uneducated about how it was transmitted, doctors were unsure of how to properly test for and treat patients, and thousands of people—many gay men among them—died within a very short span of time. The public was led to believe that the death and devastation happening within the gay community was linked to prevailing assumptions about promiscuity within this community. These were unfounded, and untrue, assumptions. As we discussed in a previous question, promiscuity is not something that is linked with a person's sexuality. AIDS, just like any other STI, is an infection that can affect any person who does not know how to engage in safe-sex practices. It's best to educate your child about STIs, no matter how they identify. As your kid becomes sexually active, it is critical that they understand the risks involved and the ways in which they can protect themselves. Because LGBTQ youth receive less instruction on these matters in school settings, it falls much more to you, the parent, to provide them with the tools they need to make safe and informed decisions. Refer to Safe Sex 101 (page 122) to help you initiate this conversation, and also look to the Resources on page 236 for further information.

Q: How do I know if someone is a friend or more than a friend?

A: The more comfortable you are with the conversations that surround dating and relationships, the easier it will be for your kid to talk to you. You won't always be able to "know" who they are dating based on behavior, but that would also be true regardless of their sexuality.

The first step is telling your child that you would like to know when they are dating someone. Explain that this isn't limited to when they are completely in love and ready to commit to a person for life; this means that if they are seeing or being physical with someone, you want to know. Make sure they know that these expectations would be exactly the same regardless of their sexuality. Without clarifying that point, your child might think that you are being more strict or harsh with them because you don't approve or don't understand. Once that is established, and you are certain that they understand that expectation, the next step is to lead with trust. If your child says that they are not interested in anyone at the moment, you have to make the conscious decision to believe them. Unless you genuinely think your child is in physical danger, you should never read their journals, talk to their friends behind their back, or pry into their personal business. Allow them to talk to you and tell you the truth about whom they are dating, and let them know that you believe what they say. Leading with that mutual respect is integral to letting your child know that you are depending on them, and they have a responsibility to be honest and upfront.

When your child does tell you that they are seeing someone, be positive. If your initial response is to ask a million questions and point out things that might not be a good fit, your child is going to walk away with a negative feeling about the experience. If there are things that concern you about someone they are dating, you can express those concerns—but don't do so in a way that makes them feel like you are trying to control the situation. They have to make their own choices, and if you are supportive of them, they will feel confident in approaching you with their own doubts and fears, and will listen more intently to your advice. By being positive, you will increase the likelihood that your child will come to you with future relationship questions.

Despite your best efforts, you may find that your child hasn't been completely honest with you. If you do discover that they have been hiding something from you intentionally, you should discuss this with them immediately and explain that it has affected your trust. This situation should be treated exactly as you would treat it if your child lied to you about a straight relationship. This is about trust, not about the gender of the person whom they are dating.

Q: How do I handle sleepovers?

A: It seemed easy enough to tell your daughter that she couldn't have boys sleep over, or to tell your son that he had to leave his door open when he was hanging out with a girl, but now that your child has come out to you, what do you do?

A great rule of thumb when deciding how to proceed is to throw gender out with the bathwater. Instead of saying that "boys can't sleep over, and girls can, but the door needs to be open," make your rules universal. A great compromise would be to say that anyone can sleep over regardless of gender, but that the sleepovers must happen in the living room or in a room where the door remains open.

Don't simply instate a rule without explaining it; have the conversation. Tell your child why you've set the rule before they have their next sleepover. These rules might make your kid feel as though you don't trust them, because you are asking them to remain in a space where they can be seen. Sleepovers are always a challenge for parents, though, even without concerns about sexual activity. Explain this to your child, and let them know that, even though you don't think they would deliberately disobey you, you would rather not be in a position that could make you both uncomfortable.

Once you make (or reinstate) this rule, don't back down. You aren't wrong. If you do think that you've made a rule too harsh, be prepared to pivot and shift the rules as you see them in action. On the flip side, if your child is leaving the door open as you asked, don't check in fifty times or come up with fake reasons to make them come downstairs. They will know exactly what you are up to, and they will feel that you're not treating them with mutual respect.

Your child may feel that you are placing these rules on them because they are gay or bisexual, and that this wouldn't be the case if they were straight. If you know they feel this way and believe it to be untrue, explain this to them, patiently, again and again. Be consistent. Your rules aren't gay rules. They are your house rules and they apply to everyone.

THE BOTTOM LINE

* Your kid's sexuality does not inform how often they engage (or want to engage) in sex, nor does it inform the emotions that they attach to having sex.

* Be open and honest about your feelings on sex. Provide your kid with the tools to make safe, informed decisions.

* Look to reliable resources to help answer your questions about sex (see the Resources on page 236 for more information). Share these resources with your child so that they will be able to look up other answers in the future.

* AIDS is not a "gay disease." Anyone and everyone engaging in sexual activity can be at risk for HIV, AIDS, and other STIs. Regardless of your child's sexuality, they need to be informed about how to protect themselves.

* Ask your child about whom they are dating, but don't barrage them with questions. Start by trusting that they will tell you if they have someone important in their life.

* Explain your rules for sleepovers, and ensure that those rules are consistent with how they were before your child came out. Your house rules needn't be specific to sexuality, and they should apply to everyone.

CHAPTER 6: Religious Beliefs

If you are a person of faith, your experience of having a gay child will likely be impacted by your religious beliefs. You may find that leaning on your faith at a time in which you are otherwise feeling confused is what helps you to stay strong and find clarity. You may, however, find that some of your beliefs are in direct conflict with this new understanding of your child. The beauty of faith is that as we grow and learn, so too does our understanding of that faith. Though your relationship to your religion may change, your faith will never be foreclosed to you, your child, or anyone in your family.

Nearly every religion hinges on love, which is the most important thing to keep as your focal point while you examine your beliefs during this time. Holding tight to your love for your child and the love that exists as the cornerstone of your religion will help enormously in guiding you as you navigate the intersections between your faith and your family.

———

Q: I'm afraid my child is going to hell.

My mom's initial response when I came out to her was not anger, but fear and sadness. She was raised in a very strict Roman Catholic family, and had been taught all of her life that people who disobeyed God would be punished for their sins. Now, here was her oldest daughter—whom she loved more than life itself—saying that she was gay. What my mom heard was nothing short of me saying, "Mom, I am going to hell." She had absolutely no idea what to do, where to turn, or how to reconcile her love for me with her fear that I would not be meeting her in heaven.

Our journey began with us fighting against each other, our eyes and ears closed. Neither of us wanted to budge on our beliefs or hear what the other was saying. Slowly, though, I began to hear her. I began to hear that she was afraid. After some time, she also began to hear me and think about how my experience might inform her beliefs. We prayed, we talked, we leaned on our faith, and we gradually journeyed together (and apart) to a new place of understanding. It isn't that my mom is never fearful about the future, but she has come to accept the things that she cannot change, and embrace the things she knows to be true. She knows that I work every day to be a kind, compassionate person, she knows that she loves me, and she knows that God loves me. Her focus is no longer set on what "might" happen, but rather on God as love.

—Kristin

A: Kristin's mother went on a very personal journey with her faith after finding out that her daughter was gay. Those who are grappling with similar struggles may have a variety of understandings of life after death, heaven and hell, or their relationship to religion itself. Some people view heaven and hell as literal, factual places. Others consider heaven and hell to be abstract ideas or metaphors. While there is no singular understanding of hell (or how one gets there), your concern most likely stems from the conflict between your unwavering love for your child and your understanding of what may happen to them in the afterlife.

In the first few days after discovering that Kristin was gay, her mother went to speak to their parish priest. She sat down with him and began to tell him what was happening and that she was scared. He asked her to pause, and said to her, "You must be a very special parent to have a child who is willing and able to talk to you about this experience. I want you to know, before you continue, that God asks us to never close our door to anyone. Not our children, not our friends, not anyone. Always listen to your child. Always keep your door open to her."

Kristin's mother has never forgotten those words, and has carried that message with her along the bumpy road of reexamining faith and religion. Most people who practice any kind of religion can agree that the most consistent message found at that religion's core is one that equates God, or a higher power, with love. Love for one another, kindness toward our neighbors, generosity, honesty, and compassion are all tenets of most religions. Hold tight to this message as you journey through this challenging time with your child.

As a spiritual person, the best thing to do when you do not—and cannot—know the answer to something is to pray, and to strive to keep an open heart and mind. Pray for guidance, pray for faith, pray for deeper understanding. Allow yourself to be open to an evolving understanding of your faith and of heaven and hell. It might not be as you thought it was, it might not be what any of us think it is, but it is certain and clear that you love your child, and you love God.

There may always be moments of doubt and fear when it comes to thinking about your child and life after death; truthfully, many of us have those concerns about ourselves and those close to us, no matter what our sexualities. Continue to love your child, and do your best to hear what they have to say. This will help you understand more about the complexities of their life, and how their experience relates to your faith. You don't have to agree with their choices completely, but the more you open your heart and mind to the knowledge that God loves your child just as much as you do, the easier it will be to continue to trust in that love and use it to help guide you on this journey.

Q: This goes against my beliefs, but I want to support my child.

A: Those are not mutually exclusive statements. You can love and support a person amid differing beliefs. What's more, belief is not necessarily a stagnant thing. The passage of time, meeting new people, and an array of various life experiences impact the way we view the world around us. Some of those moments further solidify an existing faith or set of values; others shift and reshape those views. As people, we are always learning and always re-understanding the world around us.

At this moment, you are in the midst of a journey that involves both your love for your child and how that love intersects with your beliefs. It's important to have conversations with others, paired with a readiness to learn and grow. Speak to your friends and family about your concerns and your fears, and talk to your child about these feelings as well. Ask your child how their beliefs inform and shape their understanding of themselves; remember that they also have a relationship with faith, and that their sexuality may intersect with their beliefs in many ways. You may find that your child has read up on certain aspects of their faith and can share the things that have helped them reconcile their own beliefs. You may discover that your child is feeling lost as well, and that together you can talk and look for tools to help you learn more about your beliefs and your religion.

Catalina—a Catholic who raised her children in the same faith—has a son who came out to her at fifteen. After he came out, Catalina asked many questions about her religion, examined several translations of the Bible, and found herself continually returning to the sentiment of God as love and the creator of everything and everyone. She connected this sentiment with the feeling that she and her son were both here for a reason, saying, "Maybe my son is gay so that he can help educate people about what that means. Maybe the reason I'm here is to support him. It can be very hard when you're Christian or Catholic, but ultimately, my religion is between me and God, not me and the world."

You may find that after your own exploration, you arrive at a different understanding of your faith—perhaps one that will bring you closer to your child. You may also find that this journey toward a better understanding is powerful and solidifies your current beliefs, and you may not find a way to completely reconcile your faith with your child's sexuality. That is okay. You love your child, which means that you can also respect their beliefs. So long as that mutual respect exists, there will be room for an ever-growing dialogue.

In the Resources on page 233, you'll find tools to help you develop a larger conversation around faith and sexuality. Use these resources to delve deeper into this reflective process, and to assist you in helping to better understand faith, family, and sexuality.

"We took our family to a more accepting congregation."

My son came out to us a little over a year ago. My wife and I, for some blessed reason, were able to rapidly traverse the landmine-ridden, 180-degree, whiplash-inducing evolution from actively opposing gay marriage to becoming supportive, loving parents of a gay young man. The catalyst was our son, Jordan; but the medium of our transformation was simply Christlike love. The hand of the Lord was present before Jordan came out, shaping our thoughts and preparing us. Since then, we have been guided and led from time to time, but the Lord is definitely letting us learn and grow by experience. We have also felt His hand in the new and wonderful relationships we have with many LGBT friends.

We have found that our journey is not typical. As we have become fully aware of the journey and circumstances of many others, we have begun to appreciate the hardship and difficulty of the LGBT experience. In addition, we have started to realize the complexity of understanding homosexuality and all its facets.

My wife, Wendy, and I began reaching out to family members and friends shortly after Jordan came out to us. We met with our bishop. We began meeting one by one with Jordan's youth leaders, school leaders, and people we felt would be understanding and in a position to help. We were looking for acceptance and support for Jordan as well as for ourselves.

By and large our family and community have been pretty good to Jordan. To their credit, all of our family members have treated Jordan no differently than before. Many would find this to be an unparalleled success. And to be sure, it is success; but Wendy and I have found ourselves wanting more.

Is acceptance the same as support? Jordan does very well in most social and church environments, but the more "gay" his mannerisms, the more uncomfortable and cool his acceptance gets. When we are more vocal about our advocacy for inclusion of LGBT people, we are often met with an uncommitted and profound silence. Not from those who actively oppose such things, but from many of those who profess support.

Most in our Church looked at our situation with pity, sorrow, and some sympathy, but most real support was hindered by an unwillingness to consider accepting realities outside of official teachings. Relationships I had enjoyed with church friends for more than ten years dried up and disappeared in a matter of weeks. Many expressed sadness that we were "suffering" with a tremendous challenge, but that there was really no room for compromise on perceived cultural threats. We felt very isolated within our community and I realized that the net effect was that we were being shunned.

There was no organized effort to push us out of the church, but when you collectively look down on people, the result is the same. My wife and I eventually took our family to a more accepting congregation, but I still look back with bitterness at the wasteland of long-term friendships lost. It is hard to separate the collective rejection we experienced from being rejected by God and our religious heritage. It is especially hard for my older teenage children who can't make distinctions between uncharitable members and the church itself.

My faith endures on the strength of my personal relationship with my Savior. I know He loves my son as fully today as before I knew Jordan was gay. He always knew who my son was. I don't have everything figured out, but I know that my love will be a better example to my son of my Savior's love than anything else learned in Church.

Tom, 52

Q: I want my child to be happy, but I feel that marriage should be reserved for a man and a woman.

A: There are two ways of understanding marriage: legally and spiritually. Legal marriage determines and affects legal rights such as taxes, property ownership, and health care, while marriage within religious institutions reflects a commitment as recognized in the eyes of a higher power. These are two exceptionally different understandings of one word, which is why the larger discussion around gay marriage is often very muddled. Ask yourself: Is your issue that you do not believe your child is entitled to have equal legal rights, or is your issue that you do not think that your higher power will (or should) recognize their union? Or are your religious views affecting your perspective on the legal end of things?

Marriage, in the legal sense, plays a critical part in ensuring that your child is protected. This means that should your kid ever become ill and be in a hospital, their partner will have the ability to be by their side, supporting and loving them. It means that if your child loses a partner with whom they have shared a home for twenty years, they will not have to pay taxes on the inheritance of that home. If their partner has health care, your child will also be able to receive those benefits. Legal marriage means that if your child and their partner decide to have children, they will not have to wait months, or even years, for both of their names to be legally placed on that child's birth certificate. Legal marriage is about legal rights, period.

In a religious context, marriage can mean many different things. There are certain religions that welcome gay marriage, and others that do not. Many religions will not perform certain marriages within their places of worship because they believe that their higher power would not support such a union, and, as such, neither can their congregation. This is where a personal understanding of faith enters into the picture, yet again. You may not feel that your higher power would recognize your child's union. However, your child may feel very differently, and may believe that their higher power can and will recognize the love they share with their partner. You can still love and respect your child and their partner while holding different understandings of faith.

If your kid wants to have a wedding ceremony, it won't be in a place that does not accept their union. Your child's wedding does not represent a demand that everyone adjust their religious beliefs—and this includes you. For many, spiritual marriage is about declaring love for another person in front of the people that they hold most dear, and, for some, in front of the higher power in which they believe. You can love your child and their partner, and be present as one of those people held most dear, without having to share their spiritual beliefs. You can also support your child's right to legally marry, in order to ensure that your child is protected, without having to make a final declaration on your religious views.

Just as we wouldn't fight to strip away the rights of someone who practices a different religion, so too should we feel confident in our relationship with our faith without taking away the rights of others to marry. As with anything else related to spirituality, your beliefs may change as time progresses. This is not an indicator of failure, but rather an indicator that you are growing as a person, and that your faith is growing along with you. Work to remain a consistent presence in your child's life and to not close the door to them, their partners, or their own spiritual views.

Q: How do I talk to my religious family and friends to help them understand?

A: When talking to religious friends and family, regardless of how their religion intersects with their views on sexuality, it's essential to remember that you aren't trying to get them to believe what you believe; you are only trying to communicate that you love your child. So often, when we go into discussions like these, we want to come out of them with an earth-shattering success story; we want to explain to our siblings or parents or friends that they can support a person while maintaining their faith, and we want them to believe just as we do. This isn't a fair expectation, and it's also not the only way to have worthwhile and productive communication. It is okay to have differing beliefs. When it comes to religion, there is not one "right" answer. This should be the focus of any conversation that you have with others in regard to religion:

Our beliefs are ours alone, and no one should place judgment on which ones are right or wrong.

When it comes to readying yourself for this kind of exchange, a great motto is "expect the best and prepare for the worst." There is never any telling where these conversations will lead us—sometimes the people we expect to be the most closed-minded are actually the people who help guide us through our own confusion with an open heart and mind. Sometimes the response is not as positive, and we are faced with the challenge of navigating a complex maze of Bible verses, moral tenets, and church teachings. Don't go into these exchanges expecting that you, your child, or any of the things you have to say will be rejected. That kind of expectation sets a tone that can make those responses more likely. Be open, and don't assume.

Preparing responses to specific issues that may arise will help facilitate the dialogue. If the person you are speaking with refers you to a particular Bible passage, or questions your abilities as a parent, it is good to be ready with your informed thoughts and feelings. In instances when you are being challenged, confidence in your own beliefs is often enough to guide the conversation in a relatively positive direction. There is no need to express your standpoint more than once or twice; try your best not to argue, but rather discuss your differing beliefs. Maybe the person you are speaking with will say something like, "I think it is your responsibility to push your child to turn away from this life." You can respond, in turn, with what you believe your responsibility as a parent entails. Perhaps you will say, "I understand that is your belief, but I believe that my responsibility as a parent is to love and support my child. That is what I plan to do, and I am happy to talk to you more about those decisions, but I think it is important to remember that we can both respect each other's beliefs." There are several resources, in print and online, cited at the end of this book to help you better understand various religious viewpoints. Review these materials before opening up a discussion. That preparedness will help you feel more confident with your words and help you better explain your own beliefs.

Lastly, it is important to be able to listen to the thoughts expressed by the other person, even though they may not align with your own. Just as you have fervent beliefs about your support for your child and your own faith, so, too, do others. In many instances, friends and family may cross the line and be too forceful about their beliefs solely because of how much they love your child and how afraid they are of what this may mean in the grand scheme of things. If you're willing and able to listen to these concerns, you will be able to better understand the complexities of their viewpoint. Hearing what they are saying—particularly when you may not agree—will enable a much more powerful dialogue. Respond with honesty and compassion. Tell them that you love and support your child, and your first priority is their happiness. Be willing to answer questions, and, if they express interest, offer them the same resources you have used to better understand things. Just as coming out cannot be contained within a single moment, these exchanges will not end after the first discussion. Be open to revisit these concerns, be as patient as possible, and aim to keep love at the forefront of your mind.

Q: Will my child ever have a relationship with their faith?

A: Just as your own relationship with faith has dips and bends, so, too, does your child's. Faith is a personal experience that is different for all of us, and having a relationship to a higher power or a deeply rooted belief system is not off-limits to any person based on their sexuality. There are groups within every religion that practice their faith in celebration of all individuals, and who do not pass judgment on or close doors to those who identify as LGBTQ. Scholars across the globe have written numerous books detailing the ever-shifting interpretations and analyses of different religions, and there are many places of worship that warmly welcome LGBTQ individuals. Faith is available to anyone who seeks it.

You may find that your child stopped showing interest in their faith after coming out (or perhaps even before). This isn't always a permanent shift. It is completely possible that your kid's faith will remain strong and that they just need some time to readjust or reexamine their beliefs within this new context. If your family attends a place of worship in which LGBTQ individuals are expected to change, or tells them they are not welcome, there is a chance that your child may feel shunned by their religion as a whole. This is a very valid reason for them to take a few steps back to reexamine their beliefs, but it doesn't mean that they will never return to a different understanding of that religion. They may still want to find a place of worship, but one where they feel more comfortable. Talk to your child about what they are going through. Ask them about their feelings as they relate to religion, and listen to their experience. Speak to them about your own interpretation of faith, and help them find resources that can speak to their concerns. Perhaps you had a different struggle when it came to acceptance and religion, or maybe you saw a friend go through a similar challenge. Share those experiences, and keep the conversation open.

It is important not to push your child to practice their faith in the way that you desire. Your child may navigate in and out of faith throughout their lifetime, they may find that their journey strengthens their relationship to religion, or they may find that they do not want to practice any religion at all; it is important to remember that the decisions we make when it comes to faith are not informed exclusively by our sexuality. Regardless of where their path leads them, your child needs to be given the room to explore on their own. You can certainly share your feelings, and you can invite them to go to your place of worship with you, but if they say no, it is important to allow them space. Rather than accusing or assuming ("Are you skipping church again this week?"), try saying something like, "If you would like to come to church with us, today or at any point, we would love to have you." In trying to facilitate these conversations, you may find that your child does not want to have that discussion, or share their process with you. This can be very frustrating, but know that this isn't a rejection—this is your child facing a mountain of thoughts and feelings, many of which are not easy for them to communicate. Ensure that they know you are always willing to talk, offer others who might be willing to talk to them, and remain patient.

"I'm a gay Christian."

I never expected that coming out would bring me closer to my faith, but that's exactly what happened.

Despite (or maybe because of) my very religious upbringing in the Deep South, I could never quite "click" with Christianity. I went to a massive megachurch on Sundays, then a tiny rural youth group on Wednesday nights (because a girl I had a crush on attended), and I felt like a fraud in both environments. I didn't weep during *The Passion of the Christ* like the other kids, and my heart was never warmed by the full baptisms on the Jumbotron screen above the rock-concert worship stage.

I felt disillusioned by all of the historical injustices Christianity had helped perpetrate, while at the same time, I was terrified of going to hell. Over and over I "recommitted" to Jesus, hoping to feel something. But all I felt were confusing "impure thoughts" that haunted me during morning worship, surrounded on all sides by thousands of reverent born-again Christians who I just knew would soon discover the fact that I wasn't really one of them.

Even though I couldn't connect with Christianity, I still felt fascinated by the essential mysteries of creation, human consciousness, and the afterlife. I would have checked the "spiritual, not religious" box throughout most of college and graduate school. I equated "religion" with dogma and hate, and "spirituality" with freedom and open-mindedness. Still, I longed for the ritual, symbolism, and community of church. I wanted the daily practice of religion. I understand the world through words, and I wanted a text to refer to again and again for its beauty and metaphor.

After I came out, things started falling into place. I talked to a friend's mother, who was a pastor, about alternate names for God. Instead of using the patriarchal term "Father," I could use *Holy Parent, Protector, Guardian*, or *Timeless One*. I started reading the Bible and actually enjoying it. It helped to read the text with its historical context in mind, and through a heavily metaphorical lens. Truth is not necessarily fact, and vice versa.

I talked to my partner about her experiences growing up Presbyterian— the quietness of her religion, its emphasis on service and community. She asked if I wanted to go to church with her, and I was skeptical, to say the least. So we went to a Metropolitan Community Church (a Protestant denomination with an LGBTQ outreach emphasis) and my whole world changed. Families of all types sat in the pews. Inclusive language filled the hymnbooks. Loving gay couples lined up to take communion together and then pray with one of the ministers, arms locked around each other in a tight circle. For the first time, I took communion. The whole experience moved me to tears.

Soon after, I started attending a Bible study at MCC and learned more about what it meant to be a gay Christian. These men and women viewed Jesus as a protector, a champion of the weak, the Other, the outcast. They admired the Bible's female heroes, and emphasized that there is more love and kindness in the Bible than hatred or dogma.

Sometimes people are surprised when I tell them I go to church, like being Christian and being gay are not compatible. I understand the misconception. But coming out is the reason I began re-exploring Christianity. Coming out helped me finally accept and love my real self. There were no more secrets or shame, no more lying or fear. I finally felt like I knew myself, and that meant I could open up to even more love and connectedness, this time through the framework of religion.

I'm still learning what Christianity means to me, and trying to determine how to live at peace with its troubled history. For me, it is deeply satisfying to reclaim the religion used to oppress and terrify me as a younger person. And the good news is that things are changing very, very quickly, with more and more churches of all kinds welcoming gay members, marrying gay couples, and ordaining gay clergy.

Alyse, 26

THE BOTTOM LINE

* The more you can open your heart and mind to the knowledge that God loves your child just as much as you do, the easier it will become to trust in that love and use it to help you through this process.

* Your beliefs do not have to overlap completely with those of your child in order for you to love and respect your kid. This love and respect will allow for a much-needed dialogue around your differing understandings of faith.

* Reflect on *marriage* as a word that holds two distinct meanings, one in a spiritual sphere and another in a legal sphere. It is possible to hold firm to your faith while also supporting equal legal rights for your child.

* Be open to hearing what religious friends and family members have to say, and remember that their concerns are often rooted in a place of both love and fear.

* Be patient as your child navigates a changing relationship with their faith. Remember that the journey is often what deepens and strengthens our relationship to our faith.

This Is a Book for Parents of Gay Kids

CHAPTER 7: Questioning Gender

Gender is one of the most intricate and complicated parts of self-understanding. At birth, most of us are assigned a gender based on our genitalia. Depending on our body parts, someone (most commonly a doctor) declares us a boy or a girl. That assigned gender then interacts with the dozens of layers of gender-information that we gather throughout our lives—some that we are aware of, and some that are filtered through without us noticing. Music, newspapers, television shows, magazines, children's toys, career fairs, and liquor advertisements all tell us what it *should* mean to be a boy or a girl. Infancy is painted in colors of pink and blue, and even before a child is born, studies have shown that the way people speak to the bellies of pregnant people is different based on whether the baby is going to be a boy or a girl.

There are some people who feel they fit with the gender they were given at birth, but there are also people who feel this designation does not match. Gender identity describes a person's subjective relationship to their own gender. Every person on this planet has a relationship to gender in some capacity—even if it happens to align with societal expectations in most ways. You may feel that the gender you were assigned at birth matches how you feel—this is referred to as being *cisgender*. Your child, however, might have a very different relationship to their assigned gender. They may feel that being labeled simply by their genitalia doesn't fully or accurately express their identity. They might also feel that their genitalia is irrelevant to their gender identity, and that their gender identity is based on any number of different factors. Your unfamiliarity with this process can make for a very overwhelming and confusing experience. The key here is knowledge. The more you learn about gender, and about your child's evolving understanding of their own gender, the closer you will be able to remain to them throughout their process.

In writing this chapter, we spoke to kids who were either questioning their gender or did not identify with the gender they were assigned at birth, and to their parents. The following questions, answers, and stories were inspired and informed by those conversations. We encourage you to refer to the Glossary on page 215 whenever you come across a term you haven't heard before.

———

This Is a Book for Parents of Gay Kids

Q: How is *gender identity* different from *sexual orientation*?

A: In the simplest terms possible, *sexual orientation* refers to the people you are attracted to, while *gender identity* refers to you, as a person. The gender of the person you are attracted to—romantically or sexually—is what informs your sexual orientation, while your gender identity hinges on the gender that makes you, you. For some, gender is an either/or experience—they were assigned the female gender at birth but identify as male, and may transition accordingly. For others, gender is a complex network of understandings and identity does not hinge on an either/or, but rather an exploration of what those elements mean. These individuals may identify as something outside of "male" or "female," as a combination of these gender ideas, or as constantly in shift or transition. There are many terms that are used in this conversation, all of which fall under the umbrella of *trans**. That asterisk exists as a symbol of the variety of identities and understandings within the community. Here are some common terms and definitions, which are also found in the Glossary in more detail. It's important to remember that these terms vary in meaning depending on how they are used and what they mean to the person who is using them.

- **cisgender:** A gender identity in which one's assigned sex at birth correlates with how they socially, emotionally, and physically identify (i.e., a biological male who identifies as a man is a cisgender man).

- **genderfluid:** A gender identity in which one views their gender as fluid and constantly changing.

- **genderqueer:** An umbrella identity describing someone whose gender expression or identity does not exactly align with the gender that matches their sex assigned at birth, and who views gender as more complex than either "male" or "female."

- **transgender:** A word used to describe a person whose gender identity does not match the gender they were assigned at birth.

Gender identity does not directly inform sexual orientation, nor does sexual orientation directly inform gender identity. In other words, who you are does not exclusively determine what you like, nor does what you like exclusively determine who you are. Occasionally, there may be some overlap between the two, but that is not a certain, predictable, or common occurrence. The same goes for gender identity and sexual orientation. There is no way to determine one based on the other.

Q: My child is questioning their gender. What does this mean?

A: If your child is questioning their gender, this means that they may not identify with the gender they were assigned at birth. If you've never questioned your own gender, this can be very hard to understand—so have patience with yourself as you begin to learn more about what is often a very complicated experience for both you and your child. As any child grows up, they begin to explore who they are and begin to question many different aspects of life: religion, future goals and career paths, political beliefs, cultural identity and, sometimes, sexual orientation and gender identity. Most of us struggle with some of these issues while having an easier time with others. Perhaps you never questioned the way you relate to the gender you were given at birth, but spent your adolescence exploring your spiritual beliefs, your political views, or your cultural history. The process of exploring and questioning gender is similar to these other explorations—you are reflecting on something about yourself that may or may not fit in with the concepts, ideas, and identities you had previously been given. The thing that sets the gender conversation apart from others is that it isn't as easily spoken about in many households, so these explorations can feel very isolating for your child.

Try to be as supportive as possible. No one person has the same experience when it comes to understanding themselves, and exploring something as complicated as gender is best done with people around you who support you and who are there to listen. Just as you cannot tell a person whom to be attracted to, what foods to like, what music to listen to, or what color their eyes should be, you also cannot tell a person how to identify when it comes to gender. You would likely be uncomfortable identifying as anything but the gender that you were assigned at birth (because for you, this matches how you feel)—use that imaginary circumstance as a bridge to understand that your child may be just as uncomfortable trying to "fit" the gender that they were assigned!

As with anything else, talking to your child about their process is crucial in understanding what they mean when they say they are questioning their gender. They might use terms to explain how they identify, and it is absolutely okay for you to ask for clarification on what those terms mean to them. Gender is a very personal experience, so there is not just "one" definition for most terms. Your child may come out to you as genderqueer, as transgender, or as something else entirely. If your kid is hesitant to open up and answer some of your questions, look to outside resources to become better informed about gender identity and expression. When possible, reach out to other parents who have had similar experiences—there are support groups in many communities, as well as many online communities where you can speak to others, ask questions, and share stories.

"I gave birth to a girl but raised a man."

I have a photo of my son wearing a shirt that says "(FAAB)bulous." While that means nothing to most people, for me, it stirs up myriad emotions. "FAAB" stands for Female Assigned At Birth. My son is transgender. He is male, but his road to manhood has been far more challenging than most. It has been a long road that he has not traveled alone.

My husband and I decided to have a baby right in the middle of graduate school; it seemed reasonable at the time. I gave birth two weeks after I became a Ph.D. candidate. Throughout Zak's childhood, I told people that if he had been born a boy, I would truly believe in innate gender differences; this kid was much more like a stereotypical boy than girl. He was always a free spirit, never really fitting the traditional roles for girls his age; yet he didn't fit the male mold either. While his female peers were doing their best to imitate female pop stars, he was the lone girl at local Pokémon tournaments. He was Harry Potter for Halloween in spite of how much he resembled Hermione. And oh was he upset when I wouldn't let him get a haircut like Anakin Skywalker!

We just considered him unique in every way and defended him to a world impatient for him to "act like a girl." His dad and I never cared that his gender expression didn't conform to any set societal rules. I taught him how to negotiate shopping malls while his dad did the same out in the woods.

Society tried to force him into the box marked FEMALE. His first-grade teacher worried because he spent recess playing on his own with plastic dinosaurs. Her solution to the "problem" was to have playdates with the little girls from class. I asked him if he would like that.

"No. I'm fine."

Well-meaning grandparents sent beautiful, frilly dresses. I asked him if he wanted to wear them.

"No, I just like my jeans and T-shirts."

His early teen years were fraught with emotional upheaval. There were some very low times, and I was always grateful he made his weekly counseling appointments. When he was fourteen, he told us he was a lesbian. Well, that made sense! He seemed emotionally relieved and happier. Now he could cut his hair as short as he wanted, and people accepted that he eschewed dresses and shopped in the boys' department. It was, however, a bit peculiar when he wrote a story in which the main character changed from a girl to a boy. I didn't quite know what to do with that and simply chalked it up to his remarkable creativity.

His dad and I were both accepting of his sexual orientation but handled it in different ways. I started a PFLAG group and he worried endlessly about our kid's safety. We went to several Pride events in those early years; me as a "PFLAG mom" and his dad as the protector, who'd stand back and scan the crowd for anyone who might threaten his beloved child.

College brought a whole world of new experiences, ideas, and people. By the end of his freshman year, Zak began to find the words to express his true identity. I learned all about the term *genderqueer*. For me, listening to him talk through and question his deepest sense of identity made his realization of being transgender easier to accept. I know he didn't come to it lightly.

As you would expect, his dad worried about his safety even more. I can't blame him because violence against transgender people is a sad fact of life. Transphobia is still accepted even in places where homophobia is shunned—or at least isn't expressed out loud. He worries and ruminates over the transition, but he loves our son unconditionally. As the father, he doesn't receive the brunt of the "blame" for raising a transgender child. That honor goes to me, the mother. The prevailing belief is that I was too accepting of him first being a lesbian and then being a man. I was an easy target because I did not react as expected. The typical narrative for parents of transgender children includes being distraught, ashamed, heartbroken, and inconsolable. Some of my dear "virtual" friends in my transparent support group would surely attest to that. It just wasn't my story. People close to me were concerned that I was either in denial or was pushing his transition. It was hard to express that it was neither. I didn't feel the loss of a daughter because I thought of him more as my "child" than my "daughter." Others thought that, had I insisted he accept his femininity, or at least not "gone along" with his transition, perhaps things would have been different. Of course they would have; our relationship would have been severely damaged. Not having the support and love from his family would have devastated him.

My seemingly instant acceptance of his transition made me a hero in the LGBTQ community and an enabling, negligent mother to the rest of the world. The truth is that I am neither. It isn't heroic to love your child with all your heart regardless of their sexual orientation or gender identity. It isn't negligent to allow your child to grow into their own person.

It is an emotional place to be, though: joy in my children, pride in the adults they have become, anger at those who reject the concept of transgender, rage at the violence and discrimination our transgender children face, and also awkwardness. I still feel awkward when I run into someone I haven't seen in several years and have to answer the question of how my "daughters" are doing. I know I could just brush it off with a quick "they're fine," but I can't pretend that I have two daughters.

Our son turned twenty-three this month. He is married to an amazing woman and in graduate school to become a professor, following in the footsteps of his father, his grandfather, and me. Yes, raising this wonderful young man has been interesting. A journey I wouldn't trade for anything. Only other parents of transgender children understand the daily roller coaster of emotions. Only we know how it feels when, eventually, this roller coaster slows and the ground beneath our feet finally feels solid. Only the mother of a transman can say: "I gave birth to a girl but raised a man."

Sherri, 56

Q: My child is dressing differently. Does this mean they are transgender?

I spent a long time hating the way I dressed. I didn't like when clothes fit my body snugly, and I felt weird accentuating different parts of myself. I don't know where it came from or how it happened, but I vividly remember that feeling of discomfort. It took a very long time for me to realize that what I wanted and what I wanted to want were two different things. I wanted to look good, feel good, and dress like the boys I saw on television. At the same time, though, I wanted to want my mom to think I was pretty, for my dad to think that I was cool, and for people to know that I was a girl. I get mistaken for a boy constantly, and it makes me feel so self-conscious. I'm very proud and happy with the fact that I'm female. I don't dress in boys' clothes because I want people to think I'm a boy, or because I feel like a boy. I'm just much more comfortable, and feel much more like myself in boys' clothing. I don't want to look like everyone else's idea of what a girl is supposed to be.

—Dannielle

A: From the moment we are born, we are expected to behave in specific ways based on the gender that we have been assigned. This intersects with many areas of our lives, and clothing is a central component of that behavior expectation. Although we are moving away from the time when women were expected to wear dresses and men were expected to wear slacks, we still have very strong notions of what we should or should not wear based on gender; entire department stores are divided accordingly, and advertising campaigns work to solidify this divide. The truth of the matter is this: clothing doesn't determine gender and, for many of us, gender does not exclusively determine what we choose to wear in our everyday lives. Clothing taste is one piece of a larger understanding of our identity, and though that piece may be an expression of our gender identity, that is not always (or even almost always) the case. The way we feel on the inside is not always how we choose to express ourselves on the outside and, as such, the way that your child chooses to dress cannot be used as a clear indicator of their gender identity.

If you have questions about why your child prefers to dress in a particular way, ask! This shouldn't be done in an accusatory way ("I can't imagine why you'd dress like that unless you wanted to be a girl"), but rather in a way that allows for an honest and open discussion ("Are you more comfortable in these clothes, is it a style preference, or is there something more?"). Your child's choice in dress may be reflective of style, it might be a decision based on comfort, or it could be an expression of a larger exploration of gender identity. Whatever the case, being able to express and to explore is a very important part of our identity, and being able to feel comfortable with our bodies is integral to self-esteem, confidence, and self-worth.

Keanan, who is eighteen and identifies as transgender, explained that he was always more interested in buying clothes from the boys' department, and his discomfort in women's clothing

This Is a Book for Parents of Gay Kids

increased drastically as he got older. He explained, "My mom did not understand why I felt so uncomfortable, and I didn't have the terminology to communicate those feelings. Despite how much my mom wanted me to buy clothes from the other department, I was infinitely unhappier."

Allowing your child to make clothing decisions for themselves will help them discover what makes them feel good. Your support will allow them to feel better about their journey, because they won't feel like they're doing something "wrong" by wanting to dress in the clothes marked for a gender different from their own.

It is an incredible show of support and respect for you to go shopping with your child, but only you can know what you are ready for. If you know that you will be able to go along and be supportive while helping them choose new clothes, then go, go, go! However, you may be aware that you aren't quite there yet. You may still be working to understand certain parts of your child's identity or dress, and that process may make you unable to be supportive in that specific environment. If you're concerned that you will be visibly upset while your child is picking out clothes, then you should not go along. You should, however, talk to them about your decision. Let them know that you are still adjusting to certain things, but your goal is to get to a place where you can understand them better and become more capable of supporting them. An immediate solution might be to send your child to shop with your spouse or a sibling. Regardless of whether your child is exploring a new style of dress or deeper gender issues though their clothes and style, they will need your support and acceptance. No matter what any of us say, we always want the approval of our parents. Always.

Q: How do I deal with my child wanting me to call them by a different name and use different pronouns?

A: If your child is questioning their gender, or identifies as transgender, genderqueer, or anything other than the gender they were assigned at birth, a part of their journey will sometimes involve a name change, and the request that others (yourself included) follow suit and adopt that new name and new pronouns. You may feel conflicted about this request, or upset at the thought of calling your child anything other than their birth name. You likely chose your kid's name yourself, and it's possible that you chose that name for reasons that are very important to you or your family; it might feel like they are rejecting the name you chose for them. On top of all of this, you are used to calling your child by their birth name, and you're accustomed to using certain pronouns. Being asked to change all of that can be extremely frustrating, and can sometimes feel like your kid is making things overly complicated for you and the people around them. These feelings of frustration, sadness, and confusion are understandable—this is a major shift for you, and requires patience, work, and dialogue in order to help you understand your child's perspective.

Considering your kid's perspective will enable you to be a support system as they go on this journey. It can be emotionally stressful for trans* individuals to hear their birth name and pronouns that do not align with their identity. Zak, who is a twenty-three-year-old transman, talked about this experience, saying that it felt strange to see himself one way and have the world constantly refuse to validate that view. He described the feeling of hearing the wrong name or pronouns as a feeling of rejection, saying, "It was as if they were saying, 'I don't care what you told me or what you prefer. I'm not going to listen. Your feelings aren't important to me.'" Your child may also feel uncomfortable, awkward, and nervous when you use their birth name or pronouns other than those that they prefer in public, as this sends a signal to others that they may not be the gender that they are presenting. Referring to your son in public by his female birth name can make him feel like you are telling others that he is "not actually a boy." Even in the privacy of your own home, hearing a name or pronouns that do not align with your child's gender identity can be very confusing and frustrating. Zak went on to explain that when people use the right name and pronouns, he feels human. "It is that small show of support, that linguistic nod of validation that can mean so much to a trans* person. For small words, they have an enormous impact." For these reasons, using the name your child has chosen and the pronouns they prefer is immensely important to their emotional well-being, even if you don't completely understand their need for the change.

It can be difficult to get used to this shift, and it likely won't happen overnight. After some time, your brain will readjust, and it will become second nature to use a new name or pronoun; until then, it's normal to struggle and to occasionally forget. With practice and time, it will get easier and feel more natural. In the moments when you do stumble, try not to dwell on your mistake. This is a big change for you to get used to, and it will take some time. If you accidentally use former pronouns or your child's old name, you can certainly apologize. Apologizing once is sufficient, though; making an effort, and acknowledging when you have slipped, will mean the world to your child.

Q: My child wants to use the public restroom designated for a gender different from the one they were assigned at birth. Should I let them?

A: The short answer to this question is: yes.

The longer answer involves taking many things into consideration—most important, their safety. If your child is regularly being recognized as the gender with which they identify, then it is usually safe for them to use the bathroom for that gender. Knowing what is and is not safe is, of course, very complicated. Generally speaking, it is advisable for your child to use the restroom of their preferred gender when they feel comfortable doing so, or when they feel that using the restroom of their birth-assigned gender might create an unsafe environment. Even before formally transitioning to male, eighteen-year-old Keanan would receive stares and negative or confused comments while in the women's room. "Continuing to use the women's room was starting to become an issue, and I did not want to face any larger problems such as physical harassment or the police," he explained. "I did a lot of research on how to act in the men's room, and started using it out of comfort and safety."

You and your child know your community and surroundings best, so this has to be a conversation that you have within that context. Regardless of where you live, if you think that your child may be viewed as a different gender from the designation on the bathroom they would like to use, then you should discuss the risks involved. If there is a threat of verbal or physical harassment, using single-stall, family, or gender-neutral bathrooms can be a good option. Urge your child to be aware of their surroundings, to try to avoid gendered bathrooms if the situation feels unsafe, and to bring a friend along to the bathroom when possible.

If your child is specifically asking about using restrooms at their school, then this is a slightly more complex question. School bathroom policies depend on the state you live in and the school that your child attends. Speak to the school administration about your child's bathroom situation, and try to come up with a reasonable solution based on what would work best for your child. They may prefer to use a private bathroom that's designated gender neutral (like the bathroom in the teachers' lounge or nurse's office)— but that might upset them and they may prefer to use the bathroom that matches their gender identity. Before you approach the administration, you and your child should both familiarize yourselves with the laws in your state regarding school acknowledgement of students' gender identities; you need to understand your legal rights clearly. Recent legal actions toward changing existing bathroom policies have proven successful in some cases, and there is a precedent in some areas to challenge existing discriminatory laws, if you feel inclined to do so. Look to the Resources on page 229 to help keep you current on the ever-shifting legal landscape.

In many cases, your kid is going to be the one making the decision about which restroom to enter. Speaking to them about their feelings and concerns, and ensuring that you are informed, will enable you to better understand where your child is coming from, and will also open the door to a discussion that addresses safety. The more you know, the more your child will know, which leads to the safest possible situation.

Q: My child wants to transition to a different gender. How do I handle that?

A: Transitioning means that your child is seeking to change certain aspects of themselves so they can live in a way that is more congruent with who they are, and so others can more readily recognize them as the gender that aligns with their identity. There are many different ways to transition, and no two transitions are alike. The only way to understand what, exactly, your kid means when they say the word *transition* is to ask them directly. There are several changes that can occur during a transition, most of which fall under three categories: social, hormonal, and surgical.

Social transitioning can include a variety of changes, from name and pronoun changes to wearing different types of clothes to using different bathrooms. For some, a social transition is the only transition desired. Just because your child identifies as trans* does not automatically imply that they will want to take hormones or have surgery. Again, this is why a dialogue is so crucial to your understanding.

Some transgender people feel that hormones or surgery are important components in realizing their identity, as they can help align their inner identity with their outward appearance. It is important to understand that, just as some people elect to socially transition without hormones or surgery, there are also people who elect to transition hormonally, and who never feel the need for surgery. Hormonally, estrogen can help in the development of breasts and in softening skin and curves, while testosterone can help in developing facial hair, deepening the voice, and increasing muscle mass. Surgical transitions are generally done piece by piece, and can include any number of different surgeries, ranging from rhinoplasty (nose job) to brow shaves to chest reconstruction and breast reduction to surgically altering one's genitals.

There is a marked difference in this conversation depending on whether your child is under or over the age of eighteen. If they are under eighteen, they will need parental consent to begin any form of hormonal treatment. Electing to have surgery generally requires a person to be eighteen or older. If your child is over eighteen, the decision to begin hormones or to have surgery lies entirely in their hands. In either case, it is important for you to be a part of the process. Inform yourself about the options and the changes that will occur, and make sure your child has access to the same information. The more you both know and understand about the process, the more you will be able to discuss your child's decision, their health, and the path forward.

If your child is under eighteen, it is important to work with a competent doctor who is familiar with transgender children. Puberty can be exceptionally traumatic for transgender kids. Erika Lynn said that, for her, puberty was traumatic, not because of the actual physical changes that happened to her body but because of the associations she had with those changes, and the way people treated her during that time. "It wasn't my facial hair or armpit hair that made me feel uncomfortable," she explained. "The jokes people made about how I was 'finally a man' or that I was going to start looking like a 'hairy gorilla,' or comments about how I appeared to others as more manly and masculine, was something I completely disassociated with." Because of this potential discomfort and trauma, many families choose to use hormone blockers, which hold off puberty until the child is mature enough, mentally, to give informed consent for hormone use. This will give them the time to explore their gender identity without making a premature decision. Amy's daughter, Sera, is thirteen and is currently on Lupron, which is a hormone suppresser. Amy decided to allow Sera to be on Lupron until she's eighteen, at which point she can choose whether to begin estrogen. She is under the care of an endocrinologist, so she will make that decision with her doctor. It is very rare for doctors to prescribe gender hormones for children under the age of eighteen.

Talk to your kid as much as you can about your questions and concerns, and keep an open, ongoing dialogue as things progress. If your child is uncertain, ask if they would be interested in counseling. An experienced therapist can help clarify gender identity issues for both you and your child before or as they decide to explore their options—and this is true for younger children as well. Many doctors require some guidance or confirmation from a therapist so that your child will not rush into medical decisions without careful consideration. Making sure they see a knowledgeable medical professional who has experience with other transgender patients can give you peace of mind in knowing that your child is in good hands. It can also be helpful to talk to such medical professionals about the potential risks and benefits of hormones or surgery so you know what your kid is getting into. Many parents are uncomfortable with the idea of their child making such a major change, or are afraid that hormones might be bad for their health. This is another reason why talking to an experienced medical professional can be helpful.

Talking about hormonal or surgical changes can be extremely scary for a parent since it involves a physical change to their child's body. Talk to other transgender people. This can give you an idea of what sort of changes your child will go through and what their life might be like in the future. You might be pleasantly surprised to hear how hormones or surgery have transformed some transgender people's lives; it is not uncommon for transgender people to report feeling their depression lift and to feel immensely happier through physical transition. Of course, the experience is different for everyone, but talking to others in the trans* community can give you a good idea of the possibilities for your child. Remember that the hormonal changes are very similar to a second puberty—it is not a complete personality transplant.

There will be times when you are not comfortable with a transition-related change your child wants to make. That's okay. You're not expected to be comfortable with every change immediately. However, you should do the best you can to reach a compromise. For example, if your kid would like to visit a doctor to learn more about hormone options, and you don't feel comfortable with that, find another family member or friend who could accompany them to the doctor's office. If a transition-related change is financially impossible now or in the near future, talk to your child and explain those reasons. A good compromise might be to create a long-term plan, with the ultimate goal being the completion of all of their transition-related needs.

As your child grows older, and especially after they have socially transitioned, their needs and desires may change. Transitioning is not a static, unchangeable process, but rather a dynamic journey. Your child's needs may be different at various points in their life. For example, Erika Lynn originally wanted to have a brow shave as soon as she was old enough to have one. "But after having lived as a girl for a year and a half, having a brow shave was no longer a necessity—or a desire—of mine to be happy," she says. Remember that, throughout the transition process, your child will always be your child.

"I started my transition three years ago."

I'm not one of those people who always knew I was transgender. I have friends whose earliest memories were of feeling uncomfortable with their body, and I've heard their stories of being four or five years old and feeling deeply upset at being told they were girls when they felt like boys. When I think back to my childhood, though, I don't remember having any strong feelings in general about gender. I didn't like particularly feminine things, I never liked to do my hair or paint my nails, and I was never interested in shopping for clothes. I didn't really like particularly masculine things either. I was just a nerdy, awkward kid.

There are things I look back on that seem to point toward me being trans*. I remember feeling absolutely devastated when I first got my period, and trying to ignore it in hopes that it would go away. I also had an incredibly difficult time imagining myself as a grown-up woman. Puberty was an incredibly tumultuous time for me, as it is for many people. When I was fourteen, I came out as a lesbian and things began to get better. I cut my hair short and started to dress in a more masculine way. I was from a small town and hadn't met very many gays and lesbians. I was the first out lesbian at my high school and kind of liked that people began to treat me as if I were in my own gender category. To me, that's mostly what being a lesbian was about. While I was definitely attracted to women, it was mostly permission for me to begin to look and act more masculine.

When I was eighteen, I went off to college and began to get more involved in the gay and lesbian community. I started to meet different types of lesbians, and realized that my feelings about gender were not just a lesbian thing. Later in my freshman year, I met a straight woman, and we settled into a relationship that felt surprisingly heterosexual. After we broke up, I spent some time thinking about gender, reading books by transgender people, and wondering about my own gender identity. In many ways I felt androgynous or genderless, and so for a time I considered myself genderqueer. I fell into relationships with lesbians that loved my androgynous look but were insistent that I ultimately be a woman and at least occasionally dress and act in a feminine way. This felt restrictive, but I trusted their judgment. After all, would anyone ever love me if I lived any other way?

It took a lot of reflection, therapy, and meeting other transmen for me to recognize that I did indeed identify as transgender and that I wanted to be transitioning socially. I don't know how to describe coming to that decision; it was a really long, introspective journey for me. I think that the major turning point, though, was when I met several transmen that came to visit my college for a women and gender studies conference. I spent some time with them and listened to their stories and found that we had a lot in common and that I really identified with many of the feelings they described.

Honestly, I flip-flopped a bit during this time. It was scary to come out of the closet, begin to use a new name, dress differently, and everything like that. Of my entire transition, the first few months of coming out and transitioning socially were probably the most difficult. People outright told me that they would never respect my identity, never call me by my chosen name, and never see me as a guy. Whenever I went out, people stared at me or outright asked me if I was a man or a woman. It was an extremely awkward time for me.

As I learned more, I became more interested in pursuing hormones and surgeries. I weighed the options carefully, considering my health, my future happiness, and the gravity of such a decision. I was nervous about doing anything irreversible, particularly thinking about how I would feel about such a decision twenty or thirty years from now. I was terribly uncomfortable with living in-between genders, though, and felt as though I absolutely couldn't live as a woman. I also found that I preferred the way I looked when binding my breasts and longed for a deeper voice and facial hair.

I started testosterone when I was twenty years old and had top surgery (a double mastectomy) six months later. That was more than three years ago, and I am confident that it was the right decision for me. I hardly think about gender or my coming-out story anymore, since I've so comfortably settled into things the way they are now. I live "stealth" now, which for me means that I am not open about being transgender at work or with most of my more casual friends. I am, however, much more open about these things online: I operate a blog (theartoftransliness .com) where I talk about transgender issues, and a YouTube channel where I regularly make videos about my transition.

I live my life as male now, which I suppose is strange considering how androgynous and genderqueer I considered myself before my physical transition. My feelings haven't really changed on that matter, I have just settled into being viewed as male and have become more comfortable with seeing myself that way. It's difficult to describe how I got from point A to point B; it's just been a natural thing. I recently married someone who totally respects me for who I am and we hope to some-day have children using a sperm donor. I feel confident now, I'm really happy, and I'm able to get on with my life.

Zak, 23

THE BOTTOM LINE

* Gender identity does not determine sexuality, and sexuality does not determine gender identity.

* It is possible to dress in clothes from the men's department while still identifying as female. This is specific to the person, and since gender is not only limited to being a "boy" or a "girl," intersections of dress and identity can be incredibly varied.

* Exploring identity is an integral part of growing up, and this can include clothing choices, gender expression, and gender identity.

* When it comes to changing names and pronouns, it is understandable to have a mix of emotions. Remember to view this experience from your child's perspective as well, and work to be a part of the process.

* Familiarize yourself with state laws and school policies on gendered bathroom usage. Encourage your child to gauge various situations along with their needs, and make decisions based on surroundings and safety.

→

* Changes on hormones are very similar to a second puberty, and will not result in a complete personality transplant; your child will still be the person you know and love.

* Reaching out to other parents and trans* youth who have had similar experiences will help you find answers to your questions.

CHAPTER 8: Being Supportive

If there is one takeaway you can glean from this book, it's that the most important thing you can do for your child is to continue to be a loving, consistent, compassionate parent. Your child is still your child, with many of the same needs they had before coming out to you. They should know that they can trust you and come to you in times of need, and that you love them and will remain a support system to them no matter where their life may lead. That consistency, especially in a time that can be fraught with confusion and uncertainty, will anchor them in otherwise stormy seas.

There are many powerful ways in which you can support your child. The following pages will address some specific concerns as well as more general questions. As you read, hold tight to the knowledge that your support—in whatever form it takes—will be an immeasurable source of positivity throughout your child's journey.

———

Q: My child is being bullied at school. What do I do?

A: There are several ways in which your child may be experiencing bullying. Classmates at school or people in the community may be targeting them verbally, physically, or through the Internet, or there may be various combinations of online and in-person harassment. Seeing your child go through such a difficult experience can be heart-wrenching, and many parents feel an overwhelming sense of guilt for not knowing how to make it better. If you are feeling guilty for not knowing the right way to handle the situation, know that it is unusual for a parent to be adequately prepared to handle bullying. While we wish that there were a manual given to parents of all children that helped prepare them for a multitude of things (coming out and bullying among them), that is not the reality. What's more, each child and situation is unique; there is not one answer that will solve every problem. The following gives a general overview of important things to know when your child is facing bullying, but we also encourage you to look at the Resources on page 222 so you can build upon this knowledge and seek out information specific to you, your situation, and your community.

Regardless of how you come to find out that your child is being bullied, your first step will always be to talk with them about the situation.

When you approach the conversation, keep the following in mind:

* Remain calm. Your child should know that you care about them and that the situation is important, but seeing you get extremely upset will only make things worse. It also has the potential to make your kid feel that they shouldn't come to you with these concerns (for fear of then upsetting you more), or might suggest that an inflammatory reaction is the appropriate response to the bullying itself.

* Gather the facts. No one understands the situation better than your child. Find out when the bullying began, what has happened since then, who is involved, and if any other adults have been informed or have witnessed any incidents. Is it physical, verbal, or online harassment?

* Be sensitive. Sharing information like this is often very hard, and can make your child feel very vulnerable and, at times, bad about themselves. Make sure that your child knows that this isn't their fault.

* Make a plan. Let your child know that you will not take any action before speaking with them about it, and keep that promise. Try to create a plan of action with your child so that you both feel comfortable about the way the situation is being handled.

The best-case scenario is that you and your child come to an agreement regarding the path forward. It is also possible that your child may not be willing to talk to you about the situation, or demand that you leave it alone and mind your own business. Recognize that these responses come from a variety of places—most of which are your child's feelings of insecurity, fear, and confusion. If you feel that your kid is at risk, you will have to take matters into your own hands despite their requests. It is incredibly important, however, that you listen to their concerns, remain open with them about these decisions, and explain your reasoning.

If you decide to take action, here are some suggestions:

* Talk to the school's administration. Prepare for your meeting with a list of questions: What are the school policies to handle discrimination or bullying? How have teachers been prepared? What is the administration's opinion on what should be done? Don't focus on a single incident or only your child; focus on the school as a whole.

* Engage other parents. The collective voice of many parents is a powerful force within school systems, so it is incredibly important to find out if other parents are experiencing similar issues with their children. Even if there isn't direct overlap, having them on your side can make all the difference when it comes to making change within a school. Talking to the administration from a PTA standpoint is much more powerful than speaking alone.

* Find an ally for your kid. Even if there is only one teacher or counselor at the school who understands the situation, and who your kid feels comfortable approaching, that can make all the difference. Talk to your child to see if there is someone like this at their school, and encourage them to approach that person whenever needed.

* Review school and state policies. How do those policies and state laws protect students, teachers, and schools? What can be talked about in the classroom, and what kind of assemblies can be arranged to address the issue? Several states protect teachers by allowing them to bring in age-appropriate LGBTQ curriculum without the fear of being fired. If this is the case, you will have a lot of room to suggest public speakers, books, movies, or curricula that can help encourage awareness of larger issues.

* Check in with your child. Every step of the way, communicate your plans and actions with your child. Be firm in your decisions, but also allow them to respond as things progress. You may find that an angry and silent response turns into a very vocal opinion. Listen carefully to what your child says about these situations—they often have the best feel for what is happening within school walls.

Bullying is a very complex issue and is often oversimplified to reflect a "bad person" (the bully) and a "good person" (the victim).

Keep in mind that nearly every child has been on both sides of bullying—there is a lot more at work than simply having bad kids versus good kids. Youth are taught to target those around them in many ways. The media often teaches us that we are supposed to look and act a certain way based on several factors (gender, sexuality, race, class, and ability, among others). Talk to your child about these larger issues, get them thinking about why we target each other, and always encourage them to challenge those ideas.

Q: Are LGBTQ children at higher risk for depression and suicide? What should I do if my child's behavior is concerning me?

A: Studies have shown that LGBTQ youth *are* at a higher risk for depression and suicide than their peers—but much of this research also shows that the most marked increase in these risks is found when LGBTQ youth do not have a safe or supporting home environment. It is not the genetic composition of an LGBTQ individual that predisposes them to depression and suicide, but rather a direct response to how they are treated in their communities, at school, and within their own homes. The very first thing that you should do, regardless of your child's behavior, is ensure that their home environment is safe and accepting. Be direct in your approach, and tell them, "You may find a lot of support at school and in the world, or you may find that others are

"My teacher said my bully 'probably had a crush on me.'"

The first person to ever get my sexuality right was my high school bully. I desperately hoped that my high school boyfriend would catch on when I told him that "kissing undermined our relationship." Or that my hot English teacher would reach out when I complimented her on her innovative use of shoulder pads. So when Luke chased me down the hallway, screaming, "What's up, dyke?" my first response was not, "You hurt my feelings!" but "Why, how did you know?"

Luke was an old-school kind of bully: he stole my lunch money, pushed me into lockers, and called me gay. Nothing makes a teenager feel more vulnerable than sex and sexuality. So when young people accuse each other of being gay (even in my case, where it was deeply, deeply accurate), they go where it hurts the most. Luke and I met because our gym teacher, in his infinite wisdom, decided to put us on the same volleyball team. No one ever suspected that Luke could be my bully because he was a guy and I was a girl—and those kinds of things just didn't happen. When I explained to my teacher that I was tired of Luke calling me a "little lesbian" who was "afraid of big volleyballs," he said that he "probably had a crush on me." Despite the seemingly overwhelming evidence, he did not.

My parents were the only people who noticed something was wrong. When I came home from school, I went straight from the front door directly to my room. No matter how hard she tried, my mom couldn't get me to take an interest in any of my favorite activities:

TV, talking to the dog, complaining. I was silent. Normally parents take that as a blessing, but my mom knew something was up. She began to break into my room at odd hours of the day to interrogate me.

"You're acting like you have menopause," she'd say. "God, what is going on at school?"

My mother must have asked me that same question a hundred times before I ever answered. I was afraid to tell her what was happening because I felt so ashamed. I was gay. I had a bully. I had told my teacher and I didn't know how to stop it. Still, it meant so much to me that she cared to ask, and ask a lot. "Nagging" has a bad reputation, but if my mother had never nagged me, I probably would never have told her.

When I finally told my mom, she didn't freak out. She simply sat there and asked me what I wanted to do about it. I could tell that she didn't want to know why Luke had called me gay. On a deep level, she knew: loose-fitting pants, drama-club boyfriends, celebrity girl-crushes. She wasn't yet ready to explore my sexuality with me, but she wasn't about to let me get hurt, either. I would have loved for my mother to come out and say, "Even if you're gay, it's okay." Instead she said, "He should go to jail," and it still felt so good.

We began to discuss strategy. Our plans ranged from the defensive—"Could I walk down different halls? Eat lunch in different rooms?"—to the openly aggressive—"Should we inform the teacher? The principal? His dumb girlfriend?" Throughout the process, my mom didn't take one step without talking with me first and getting my consent.

My mother decided not to hit Luke with a truck, but to instead come into the school and form a coalition of parents who were concerned about harassment. It may not have been a Gay-Straight Alliance, or a

PFLAG, or a chapter of Amnesty International, but it was a group of people saying something about the issue. I'm not sure what they did besides meet twice a month and scream at the principal about the terrible kids in his school. I do, however, remember the feeling of seeing those moms walk past security and storm into his office, demanding attention and justice and more pizza in the cafeteria. It made me proud.

Something about what my mother did inspired me to action. I cried in my gym teacher's office until it made him so uncomfortable that he had no choice but to put me on another volleyball team. When Luke would point at a random girl in the hallway and ask me if I liked her, I would tell him I didn't need her—I already had his sister's number. I refused to give him my lunch money. I told other teachers that he upset me. And on the last day of school, I hit him in the face with a volleyball. I knew my mom was watching.

Heather, 28

less welcoming. I want you to know that no matter what happens outside of this house, you will always find support here." Reinforce that message at every turn.

If you notice a change in your child's behavior, however slight (perhaps they have stopped seeing friends, they have been staying in their room much more often, or they don't seem to take any interest in their old hobbies or activities), ask questions. Is something happening at school? Are they fighting with friends? It can be exceptionally difficult to talk to your child when emotions are high, and you may meet with a negative or resentful response. Your kid's reluctance may make you feel that the best thing to do is to back off. While you shouldn't barrage your child with constant questions, it is also important to remember that being in the emotional place of a teenager might result in screaming, complaining, and pushing you away, but it doesn't stop your child from needing you. Keep encouraging them and asking questions. Keep showing up at their intramural soccer games, keep asking how their day was, and keep eating dinner together. In situations that do not seem life-threatening, being a consistent and supportive parent is often the best thing that you can do. This may also be an excellent opportunity to see if they would like to see a counselor. Sometimes it is much easier to open up to someone other than a parent, and that option should always be on the table.

If you notice a severe shift in behavior, or are concerned about your child's well-being, counseling is highly encouraged. The

Resources on page 232 will help you find social workers and therapists who are sensitive to and experienced with LGBTQ issues. Even if your child's troubles aren't rooted in sexuality or gender identity, specifically, it is still important that they speak to someone who is familiar with these issues. Know that there are many different options for counseling depending on your financial position, as well; especially for youth, there are often incredible counseling options available for little to no cost. You might also want to consider going to therapy together. You can explain to your child that you have concerns and questions about how best to handle certain situations. Family therapy will enable you to work on your communication with your child, and will also give both of you a much-needed outlet for talking about your feelings. If your child prefers to go to therapy without you there, let them. Counseling is a great way to find a third-party perspective. Oftentimes, being in the middle of an experience makes it very difficult to see possibilities for solutions or for change, and even if your kid goes alone, it can still be incredibly effective.

If your child is acting in a way that is self-destructive, causing themselves physical harm, or speaking actively about harming themselves or others, seek help immediately.

UNITED STATES SUICIDE HELPLINES

✳ **The Trevor Project Lifeline:** 866-488-7386

✳ **National Suicide Prevention Lifeline:** 800-273-8255

Q: Should I become more politically active now?

My dad isn't the kind of person who will hold signs up on the side of the road in support of my rights; he didn't join PFLAG and he never got "Big Gay Daughter Dad" tattooed on his arm (mostly because he's afraid of needles), but he's always been supportive in his own, unique way. He is the kind of person who will voice his opinion if the situation arises, but who doesn't seek those situations out. He's not one to push his beliefs on others, but he will absolutely stand up for equality and against prejudice when necessary. I am the way I am because of his presence in my life. I don't think you have to spend every waking second "fighting for rights" in order to fight for rights. You make your own way with it.

—Dannielle

A: When it comes to being politically active as the parent of an LGBTQ child, do what makes you comfortable. There is no obligation to get involved on a political level—but if that is where your heart is pulling you, it's a remarkable role to fill.

You may feel moved to action now that you are armed with more information about LGBTQ youth, or the LGBTQ community at large. First, think about what you mean when you say "politically active." Are you frustrated because you think there should be more support on the local or school level for your child and other LGBTQ children? Do you want to become more educated about local, state, and national representatives so that your vote can be better informed? Would you like to help implement new or improved policies on a larger scale? Do you want to run for office? There are so many forms that political involvement can take, and some may feel more comfortably aligned with your personality and your interests. If you aren't confident speaking in front of others but feel that you'd like to voice your opinion, you can write letters to editors, start a blog, compose a song, create art that sends a message, or do various other things that utilize your skills and interests in a way that also is active and political.

If you are not moved to take action outside of simply being a supportive and informed parent, that is not only acceptable—it is commendable. Many might argue that it is also, in its own right, a political act. Don't ever let others make you feel that you should live or behave in a way that doesn't feel comfortable to you simply because you have an LGBTQ child. Some of us have a fire that needs to be acted upon in a public manner, and others have a passion for things that we address in more nuanced, personal ways. In order for you to be a good parent, you also have to do the things that align with who *you* are. Even if you don't want to increase your political involvement at this point in time, having knowledge about political candidates and voting in your local, state, and national elections is an extremely powerful way to share your voice.

If your kid wants you to attend events and become more involved and you're not sure how that will make you feel, try some new things before you make a final decision. We interact with parents all the time who bring their child to Pride celebrations, drive them to LGBTQ events, and help them become and remain involved in the community in various ways. There are many levels of showing your support and becoming an active member of the community, so there is certainly a way for you to navigate those options with your child. The effort you put toward trying new things will mean the world to them, and along the way you will also learn more about yourself and your interests.

Don't feel obligated to throw yourself into the political deep end right away. Take things one step at a time. Perhaps you will go to the next Pride celebration in your town or in a nearby area. Maybe you will reach out to a local PFLAG chapter and begin by talking to other parents about their involvement. It is possible that this step might lead you to gather signatures for a local campaign or petition. That could inspire you to compose and send a letter to your local government asking for specific changes in a county-wide school policy. You may find that none of these things align with your interests, but at least you tried!

If you want to find more ways to become active in your community, look to the Resources on page 222 for organizations that will be able to help guide you.

Q: **My political party does not actively support LGBT rights. How can I reconcile this?**

A: Many factors go into choosing a political party (or particular political candidate), and there are many critical issues to be considered. You are not obligated to vote for a candidate

"We wanted to be active in the community."

My wife, Catherine, is a real type-A, take-charge kind of person. She and I had had a couple of conversations about our son, Michael—I think she knew that he was gay but was so frustrated that he hadn't told us. She wanted to hear it from him. I kind of had an idea, too, and Catherine and I had talked for several days ahead of time before she eventually grilled it out of him.

I was downstairs at the time, and Catherine came down and said, "Hey, Michael wants to talk to you up in his room." I felt like I knew what was coming. So popped up to his room, and I remember he was lying on his bed. I said, "What are you going to tell me? I think I know, but go ahead and tell me." Then he said, "Hey, Dad, I just—I want to let you know that I'm gay." There was no small talk—he just laid it right out there. I gave him a big hug and asked him a few questions. I can't say it was a big stunner for me, so I wasn't speechless or without words. I don't think I was caught off guard like some parents might be.

Catherine and I tend to be centrists in our political views. We're fiscally conservative, but we have always been very socially progressive. Our political inclination has been mostly supportive—and in the worst cases, tolerant. After Michael came out as gay, though, we really embraced activism. We immediately got involved. Catherine was instantly reaching out on the Internet and compiling support resources. I think it's something that's in our DNA—not to want to control, but certainly to lead, and to set the pace.

One of the most memorable moments for me was a rally on the steps of the Custom House in downtown Charleston, South Carolina, on a chilly March day. It was a wonderful event. Even though Michael was out of town, we were still there to support him. Catherine and I went with a number of members of the safe-space group that he attends, and it was just a great, open meeting. There were no protesters, nothing ugly about it, just a very positive message of love and solidarity.

So now we're going to go to the rallies, we're going to get out in front, and we're going to cheerlead when that's the best that we can do. We are making our choices more on the socially progressive and socially supportive side, and that's becoming the primary determinant of how we'll vote and what we'll fund. If you can lead the way, that's good.

Michael, 42

with a long track record of gay-friendly policies simply because you now have a child who may be directly impacted by them. However, you *do* have an obligation to understand the implications of those policies (or lack thereof) and how those weigh against other relevant topics.

Many of us think that we need to choose and adhere to one political party across the span of our lifetime, and that we also must agree with that party's positions across the board. It can often feel like we aren't voting on specific issues at all, but rather that we are voting for one person to accurately express our opinions on everything. That is a seemingly impossible task. You may find that a candidate aligns with your views on foreign policy, education, the environment, and immigration (all incredibly important issues), but that you disagree with that candidate's position on marriage equality and gun control (also extremely important issues). Make a list of the things that are meaningful to you, and then prioritize that list. Base your vote on what matters most to you. There is a chance that a politician who votes against gay marriage may work to pass another law that has an exceptionally positive impact on education, immigration, or health care. Only you can decide what matters most and, though it may be difficult, you have to be able to answer to yourself at the end of the day. If you know why you have made your decisions, you can then share your thoughts with those who question or challenge your reasoning.

Speak to your child about your process. Let them know the work that you put into coming to your conclusions and decisions.

Ensure that they know you support them in many ways, and that you are also willing to dialogue about how your political interests may be conflicted. Be willing to hear how they feel about the issues. You may find that your discussion with your child and your exploration of your opinions lead you to a place where you change your party stance. It may be a gradual shift, it may happen immediately, or it may not happen at all. Let an equal measure of head and heart guide you. We all make decisions based on various factors, and many of them weigh differently on our minds depending on who we are and how we experience the world. You may also find that your child will start weighing other factors beyond gay marriage and rights into their own political decisions. You and your child both stand to learn a lot from this experience, even if the road forward isn't always perfectly paved.

Q: Should I join support groups?

I never, ever thought that my mom would be the kind of person who would look to a support group to talk about my sexuality, so it came as a very big surprise to me when, about three years after coming out to her, I found a PFLAG pamphlet tucked in the back seat of her car. When I brought the pamphlet to her attention, she replied enthusiastically, "Oh, yeah! Have you heard of The PFLAG? They came in to talk to people at my job and I told them all about you!" Trying to conceal my amusement at her calling the organization "The PFLAG," I asked what she had thought of the experience. She was, with no exaggeration, ecstatic. She had asked one of the young women tons of questions about her life, how she knew she was gay, how her parents felt about her being gay, and the list went on. After that initial experience, my mom began talking to other people in the community who were gay or who had gay children. As she gathered more information from those around her, she seemed to get increasingly comfortable asking me questions. I think that one experience with PFLAG was a real turning point in her journey.

—Kristin

A: You should absolutely join support groups if that is something that feels right to you, personally. You are certainly not required to—though many parents do find a wonderful community by doing so. The best thing to do at this point is to better understand what support groups offer, get a general sense of what it's like to attend one, and then use those guideposts to inform how you would like to proceed.

What they look like: Support groups like PFLAG (Parents, Families and Friends of Lesbians and Gays), or meetings held at local LGBTQ Community Centers, are open to the public. Some meetings are only for the parents and friends of LGBTQ youth, while others (often referred to as "mixers") are open to families, friends, and the youth themselves. It will vary from place to place, but support groups generally involve a circle of chairs where everyone who attends can sit and talk with each other. Most meetings begin with everyone introducing themselves and possibly saying something about their week. No one is forced to speak about their child if they aren't ready, and participants can be as vocal or as quiet as they wish. There is usually a moderator who guides the group through a list of conversation points. These might include topics as complex as religion and sexuality, or as simple as your opinions on curfew times for teenagers. Most meetings like these are designed to bring people together around points of commonality, and topics of conversation are often suggested by members. Meetings are held in common spaces such as meeting halls, churches, libraries, or even people's homes; they are free of charge, and the organization operates under a confidentiality policy. What is said during the meetings and whoever attends the meetings remain private.

What they offer: The beauty of sitting with others in your community who may also have LGBTQ children is that you will find others who are having (or have had) experiences similar to your own. Just as it is damaging for LGBTQ youth not to see others who are facing the same questions and concerns as them, so, too, can it be damaging for you, as a parent, to be unaware that others have the same questions as you. Support groups offer a space where you can be yourself without having to fear judgment. The premise of support group meetings is to create a welcoming place for those who might feel too scared to share their questions with others.

Sergio, whose son Daniel recently came out to him, said that a huge step in his process was finding other families going through a similar experience. "Now, if I know of someone who may have a child that is gay, I want to help," he said. "I want them to know they can come to us, and we can help them understand that their child is still their child." Groups like PFLAG offer you the chance to meet people who can understand your concerns, remind you that others have gone through similar situations, and also offer you ways to find further support, should you need it. The conversations that you have both within and outside of these meetings can help you better understand your feelings, and can help you prepare for what's ahead.

If all of that sounds like the best thing you've heard of since sliced bread, then you should absolutely go to a local support group meeting. You might also feel that you have a sufficient community in your friends and family, or that you would rather deal with your emotions in a way that doesn't involve sitting in a room with others. Not going to a PFLAG meeting doesn't equate with not supporting your child. In fact, as this chapter has hopefully illustrated, you can support your child in many ways without joining a support group; however, joining support groups is an optional way to support *yourself*.

Also, perhaps you will want to seek out a support group, but now just isn't the right time. Heading to a place like PFLAG may sound horrible to you today, but in three months may be exactly what you need to take that next step. It is possible that you will feel uncertain, and venture to a meeting to see what it is like; you may find that trying it out was the best decision you ever made, whether it led you to discover that you love the meetings or that you'd rather not return for more. If you decide to attend a meeting, you don't have to go alone. It is completely acceptable to bring a close friend or family member along with you, even if they just accompany you to the first few meetings so you can find your comfort zone. There is no way to mess up looking for support.

We've spent the entire book telling you to support your child and help them to find happiness, but it is equally (if not more!) important to also take care of yourself. You can't be a supportive parent without knowing what you want and how you're feeling. There are several resources available to you (many of which are listed in the Resources on page 222) that can supplement work in support groups, or stand on their own.

Q: **How can I show my pride without embarrassing my child?**

A: Follow the cardinal rule: Do not paint your entire living room in rainbow colors or dye the dog's fur purple.

In all seriousness, having pride in your kid and in the LGBTQ community as a parent of a gay child is a brilliant thing. Know that your intentions are valued and your pride has (and deserves) a space. But your pride may be different from your child's, and it is important to be respectful as well as proud.

There is a large scope of identity within the LGBTQ community. Some of us like to wear rainbow leotards and feather boas, cover our bodies in glitter, and march in Gay Pride parades across the globe. Some of us don't identify as much with the larger

LGBTQ community, and don't feel compelled to define or mark our identity by participating in activities with other LGBTQ individuals. There are also those of us who fall somewhere in between; we love to attend Pride celebrations and enjoy feeling a part of a larger community on occasion, but on a daily basis we shake off the glitter and simply feel like human beings. The same goes for parents, friends, and family of LGBTQ youth. Since there are many different ways that we all engage with being "proud" of who we are, there is a chance that you aren't on exactly the same page as your child.

Buying lots of rainbow flags or T-shirts from LGBTQ organizations might be your way of saying, "I support what you do! I love you! This is great!" However, this is not your journey to go on alone; it is your journey to go on *with* your child. Start by telling your child that you are proud of them—so proud, in fact, that you want to get involved with the LGBTQ community on a bigger level. Their first response might be, "Oh my God, Mom, please. No. Don't. Just. Can't you please just stay home?" Let them know that you are not going to go out of your way to embarrass them or expose their sexuality to people who are unaware of it. Explain to them that you being involved does not have to interfere with the way they live their life, and tell them, "Because I love and support you, I need to have the ability to express my support in my own way. *Capeesh?*" (You don't have to say capeesh, but can elect to if you are Italian or just generally feeling it.) Your child needs to know that you having pride doesn't mean you will drag them along to a million events where they give out free beaded necklaces. You are entitled to make your own choices, but be careful not to interfere with their process.

If your kid doesn't want you flaunting your pride while they are in earshot, begin by finding a group that you can join on your own (or with a friend or other family member). Community centers or groups like PFLAG provide fun ways to become more involved with the LGBTQ community. Not only will those resources allow you to show your pride and support, but they will also give you a network of other proud parents who have similar interests. This means that if your child doesn't want you to go along with them to the Pride parade, you have a built-in community to look to for companionship. Sure, your kid might duck under the nearest tree when you come parading down in your feather boa, but you gave them the space that they needed, you are expressing your pride, and, if they don't already, they will eventually come to appreciate your support (and your boa).

THE BOTTOM LINE

* Your support—in whatever form it takes—is and will continue to be a vital part of your child's journey.

* If your child is being bullied, ask them questions, get information, create a plan with them when possible, and keep them in the loop on your plan when you think they may be at risk.

* When talking to school administration about bullying issues, know school and state policies, work with other parents to present a united front, and focus on the school as a whole instead of on one specific incident.

* You arc not obligated to become more politically active, but should you feel compelled to do so, there are many incredible ways to get involved in your community.

* Negotiating political party stance doesn't always mean one thing. Create a list of your priorities when it comes to voting, and discuss these with your child.

→

* Support groups provide a strong community of people who share similar experiences, but your participation is entirely dependent on your interest and your needs.

* Showing pride in your child and the LGBTQ community is commendable; it is also possible to do so while being respectful of your child's wishes.

This Is a Book for Parents of Gay Kids

➜ MOVING FORWARD

You did it!

You read the entire book, or you skipped to the back to see if there was a one-sentence way of answering all of your questions. Spoiler alert: There is not a magic sentence, so if that is how you landed here, you should probably go back and read the book. For the rest of you, it is pretty wonderful that you dedicated the time to better understand what's going on in your kid's head, what's going on in your own head, and how to bring those two things together in the best way possible.

Hopefully, what you have read here has shined a light on the importance of dialogue, patience, and reflection. An honest and open dialogue is key at this juncture in your family's life. While your child may not be at a place to engage with that dialogue right this moment, that doesn't mean you can't seek out information on your own time while they continue to work through their own concerns. Having patience is incredibly important, both with your child and with yourself. Your child is likely working to understand themselves, or to become comfortable within a new understanding of themselves—this takes time. Simultaneously, you are also working to adjust to a new reality. In some instances, that might be an easy task; in others, it can be exceptionally difficult. You are no better or worse of a parent if your journey takes you more time than that of the next guy. We all walk different paths, and the important thing is that they lead toward understanding and love.

A lot of people don't give parents enough credit for the work they put in to facing the challenges inherent in their kid's coming-out process. This is also *your* coming-out process. So much attention is placed on helping the kid, caring for the kid, supporting the kid, and, while this is very deserved attention, it's sometimes forgotten that you, as the parent of that kid, need support as well. More than support, you need encouragement. More than encouragement, you need appreciation. Know that you are appreciated.

So, thank you. Thank you for being an incredible parent.

Glossary

While we know that a glossary is of the utmost importance for a book such as this one, please understand that we are not the rulers or creators of LGBTQ vocabulary. Many of the words you will find below are terms for complicated concepts, and this list is by no means exhaustive. Words, especially labels, are self-defined. Two people with very similar sexual orientations or gender identities may identify with two different words. We have defined these words to explain their meaning on a basic level, but if you are curious about additional vocabulary or are still confused, more resources are available. You can start with those at the back of this book.

ally: An individual who does not identify as LGBTQ but supports the LGBTQ community, or works with and for the LGBTQ community to advocate social and political issues.

androgynous: A term for an individual who doesn't appear to be distinctly "masculine" or "feminine." Androgyny can be physical, expressional, or both.

asexual: Those identifying as asexual are not sexually attracted to anyone. Asexual people often experience romantic attraction and may choose to engage in romantic relationships.

binding: Binding involves using an elastic binder, bandages, or tape to bind one's breasts tighter to the chest. This is often done by trans* individuals to help them pass as male.

biphobia: Fear, ignorance, intolerance, and other negative attitudes and actions directed toward bisexual and pansexual individuals. Biphobia can also be experienced, intentionally or not, within the LGBTQ community.

bisexual: Someone who is capable of being attracted to many genders. (*See also* pansexual.)

cisgender: A gender identity in which one's assigned sex at birth correlates with how one identifies socially, emotionally, and physically (e.g., someone who was assigned male at birth who identifies as a man is a cisgender man).

closeted: The status of an LGBTQ-identified person who has not told others that they are LGBTQ. One can be closeted to everyone, to most people, or to only a specific group of people (e.g., closeted to one's family but out to friends).

coming out: The process of an LGBTQ person voluntarily telling other people that they identify as LGBTQ. This is different from "being outed," in which someone else reveals your identity without your consent.

cross-dressing: Expressing one's gender differently from that of one's assigned sex with clothing, makeup, hair styling, binding, etc. The term *cross-dressing* is usually used by cisgender people, as transgender people do not feel they are "cross" dressing but rather dressing to reflect the gender with which they identify. Because of this, cross-dressing is a term that can be interpreted as derogatory or ignorant when used to describe transgender people.

drag king: A woman who dresses to appear as a man, often for an act or performance. A drag king might express their gender as masculine in their everyday life but does not necessarily identify as trans*.

drag queen: A man who dresses to appear as a woman, often for an act or performance. A drag queen might express their gender as feminine in everyday life but does not necessarily identify as trans*.

FTM (F2M): A female-to-male transgender or transsexual person. One does not need to have undergone surgery to identify as FTM. FTM is synonymous with the term *transman*.

gay: A word used to describe a person whose sexual and/or romantic orientation is toward those of the same gender.

gender: While gender is generally assigned at birth, along with sex, it also houses a much broader range of issues related to physical appearance, expression through clothing, activities, and behaviors.

gender expression: The way in which one dresses and/or acts in society that is often categorized on the masculine/feminine spectrum. Gender expression is connected to gender identity, but one's gender identity cannot be assumed from one's gender expression (i.e., a person may dress in a more "masculine" or androgynous manner, but identify as female).

genderfluid: A gender identity in which one views one's gender as fluid and constantly changing.

gender identity: An individual's self-identification along the gender spectrums. Gender identity can include one's sex (man, woman, intersex), one's identification of their sex (*transman, transwoman*), one's location on the masculine/feminine spectrum, and one's attitude toward gender (genderqueer, gender fluid, etc.).

gender-neutral pronouns: Various pronouns that are used by gender-nonconforming people to avoid the gender binary of only "he/his" and "she/her."

genderqueer: An umbrella identity describing someone whose gender expression and/or identity does not exactly align with the gender assigned to them at birth.

GSA (or QSA): A middle school, high school, or college club that stands for Gay-Straight Alliance or Queer-Straight Alliance. GSAs range in activities and purposes, but generally provide a space for support, advocacy, and social interaction.

heterosexism: Attitudes, bias, and discrimination that favors heterosexuals. This can include making the assumption that others are heterosexual, or that being heterosexual is the "norm," or is superior to other sexual identities.

heterosexual: A person whose sexual and/or romantic orientation is toward those of the "opposite" gender.

homophobia: Fear, ignorance, intolerance, and other negative attitudes and actions directed toward LGBTQ individuals (*also see* biphobia *and* transphobia). Homophobia ranges in intensity, from subtle exclusion to bullying to hate crimes.

homosexual: A person whose sexual and/or romantic orientation is toward those of the "same" gender.

intersex: A word used to describe people who are born with both male and female sex markers (genitalia, hormones, chromosomes). There are at least sixteen ways to be intersex. Many intersex infants are surgically or hormonally treated by doctors to align all sex markers with either the male or female sex, sometimes causing later developmental problems. The term has replaced *hermaphrodite*, which is considered offensive.

lesbian: A gay woman. Some identify with the word, while others identify more strongly with other labels, such as gay or queer.

LGBTQ: An acronym that stands for lesbian, gay, bisexual, transgender, and queer/questioning. This acronym has many variations and additional letters that are often added to represent intersex, allies, and other identities.

This Is a Book for Parents of Gay Kids

MTF (M2F): A male-to-female transgender or transsexual person. One does not need to have undergone surgery to identify as MTF. MTF is synonymous with the term *transwoman*.

pansexual: Someone who is attracted to people regardless of gender. Pansexual and bisexual people alike often operate with a nonbinary view of gender, meaning that they are attracted to people who do not identify as strictly male or female.

pass: A term most often used among the trans* community to describe when an individual is viewed ("passes") as the gender with which they identify, rather than as the gender they were assigned at birth.

PFLAG: Parents, Families and Friends of Lesbians and Gays. Founded in 1972, PFLAG is a non-profit based in the United States that serves as an ally advocacy organization, as well as a support network for families and friends of LGBTQ people.

physical transition: The process by which a trans* person transforms their body to reflect their gender identity. This can include hormone injections and/or surgery.

Pride: A term used often in the LGBTQ community to refer to people's celebration around being LGBTQ. Many communities hold Pride events to highlight LGBTQ accomplishments, and to show unity and happiness surrounding all sexual and gender identities.

queer: An umbrella term often used to refer to anyone who is not heterosexual and/or cisgender. Some people, especially those in older generations, still find the term offensive, while others find it empowering. "Queer" is also used in academia in a broader sense as a means of discussing behaviors, trends, and identities that fall outside of societal expectations or norms.

sex: One's categorization as male, female, or intersex at birth based on sex markers such as genitalia, hormones, and chromosomes.

sex-reassignment surgery: Also known as a sex-change operation in popular culture, it is an operation that physically changes one's genitals through plastic surgery. Sex-reassignment surgery is the preferred term for this operation by many in the trans* community.

sexuality: A term sometimes used interchangeably with sexual orientation. In reality, *sexuality* is a word that also includes other attributes, including one's sexual orientation, biological sex, gender identity, and sexual practices.

sexually transmitted infections (STIs): Infections that have a significant probability of being transmitted between individuals by means of sexual behavior, including vaginal intercourse, oral sex, and anal sex. The term has come to replace STDs (sexually transmitted diseases) because *infection* is considered a less stigmatizing term since many STIs can be treated.

sexual orientation: A term used to describe one's sexual, affectional, emotional and/or romantic attraction. Words used to describe one's sexual orientation include *homosexual, heterosexual, bisexual, pansexual, asexual, gay, straight,* and *queer,* among others.

social transition: The process for a trans* person of shifting from one gender to another without surgery or hormones. This can include coming out and/or changing one's hairstyle, clothing, pronouns, name, activities, etc.

straight: A word used to describe a person whose sexual and/or romantic orientation is toward those of the "opposite" gender. A more commonly used word than "heterosexual."

trans*: An umbrella term used to describe all people who are gender nonconforming. This can include, but is not limited to, transgender people, transsexual people, and other gender-nonconforming identities. The asterisk is used to refer to the many different identities that are all a part of the gender-nonconforming community.

transgender: A person whose gender identity does not match the gender they were assigned at birth.

transition: The process a trans* person undergoes to shift from their assigned sex at birth to the gender that is aligned with their gender identity. One's transition can include both a social and physical transition.

transphobia: Fear, ignorance, intolerance, and other negative attitudes and actions directed toward those who do not identify and/or express their gender in a way that, according to social conventions, "matches" their assigned sex. Transphobia is targeted at those who do and do not identify as trans*.

transsexual: A word used to describe a person who identifies with a gender different from the one they were assigned at birth. Transsexual people usually, but not always, pursue a physical transition that includes hormones and/or surgery. Sometimes, prefixes are added to the word *transsexual* to indicate if and/or when the person will have surgery—*pre-op transsexual* means they are planning to have surgery, *post-op transsexual* means they have had surgery, and *non-op transsexual* means they have no intention of having surgery.

Resources

FAMILY AND PARENTING

Family Acceptance Project

familyproject.sfsu.edu

This project focuses its efforts on how a supportive family can greatly decrease the risks for LGBTQ youth. It conducts research, education, and policy initiatives, and offers intervention and counseling.

PFLAG (Parents, Families and Friends of Lesbians and Gays) National Office

202-467-8180

www.pflag.org

The nation's largest family and ally organization. Made up of parents, families, friends, and straight allies united with people who are LGBTQ, PFLAG is committed to advancing equality and societal acceptance of LGBTQ people through its threefold mission of support, education, and advocacy.

The Parents Project

www.theparentsproject.com

A website that is dedicated to providing advice, video content, and resources to parents of LGBTQ youth.

Bullying

Gay, Lesbian, and Straight Education Network (GLSEN)

www.glsen.org

National education organization that works to ensure safe schools for all, regardless of sexual orientation or gender identity/expression.

Safe Schools Coalition

Crisis hotline: 877-723-3723

www.safeschoolscoalition.org

An international presence that offers information, resources, and skill-based training for students, educators, and community members seeking to create safer schools for LGBTQ youth.

Stop Bullying

U.S. Dept. of Health & Human Services

Lifeline: 800-273-8255

www.stopbullying.gov

A U.S. government website that hosts information from various government agencies about bullying and cyberbullying.

Ambiente Joven

www.ambientejoven.org

Specifically for Spanish-speaking LGBTQ youth, an online resource that covers topics such as coming out, STIs, and local resources.

Everyone Is Gay

www.everyoneisgay.com

An LGBTQ youth organization founded by the authors of this book that provides online advice, videos, and resources, and offers an ongoing presence at high schools and universities.

I'm from Driftwood

www.imfromdriftwood.com

A collection of online videos described as "true stories from gay people all over."

It Gets Better Project

www.itgetsbetter.org

An organization and online move-ment that works to inspire needed change and hope to lesbian, gay, bisexual, and transgender youth around the world.

Youth Guardian Services

877-270-5152

www.youth-guard.org

A youth-run nonprofit whose main service is Youth Talk Lines: group e-mail lists that connect LGBTQ and straight supportive youth to talk with each other about anything in a safe space.

Books for Young Children

And Tango Makes Three, by Justin Richardson and Peter Parnell. New York: Simon & Schuster Books for Young Readers, 2005.

Roy and Silo, two male penguins, unsuccessfully try to start a family until they are given an egg by a zoo-keeper and thus hatch their own daughter.

The Family Book, by Todd Parr. New York: Little, Brown Books for Young Readers, 2010.

All sorts of families are depicted in this book, including ones that can have two moms or two dads.

The Harvey Milk Story, by Kari Krakow. Ridley Park, Pennsylvania: Two Lives Publishing, 2002.

A picture book biography of important gay-rights figure Harvey Milk.

My Princess Boy, by Cheryl Kilodavis. New York: Aladdin, 2011.

A story about a little boy named Dyson, who loves pink, sparkly things, and wears dresses as well as jeans.

Books for Teens

The Full Spectrum: A New Generation of Writing About Gay, Lesbian, Bisexual, Transgender, Questioning, and Other Identities, edited by David Levithan and Billy Merrell. New York: Knopf Books for Young Readers, 2006.

Written by a variety of LGBTQ teens and young adults, this anthology of narratives and stories describes many of the possible experiences of growing up as an LGBTQ person.

GLBTQ: The Survival Guide for Gay, Lesbian, Bisexual, Transgender, and Questioning Teens, by Kelly Huegel. Minneapolis: Free Spirit Publishing, rev. ed., 2011.

Frank information and advice for teens who are questioning their sexuality or have already come out. Topics include coming out, getting support, and the current LGBTQ rights movement.

Queer: The Ultimate LGBT Guide for Teens, by Kathy Belge and Marke Bieschke. San Francisco: Zest Books, 2011.

A comprehensive guide for LGBTQ teens about issues ranging from coming out to relationships to sex, written by two well-known queer authors.

National Center for Transgender Equality

www.transequality.org

Leading organization that focuses on legal rights for transgender people.

Websites

The Art of Transliness

theartoftransliness.com

Advice and resources for trans youth.*

The Gender Book

www.thegenderbook.com

An online book that explains gender in an inclusive and comprehensive way; accessible for any age.

TransHistory

www.tghistory.org

An interactive timeline of transgender history, beginning with the third century.

Books

Transgender 101: A Simple Guide to a Complex Issue, by Nicholas M. Teich. New York: Columbia University Press, 2012.

Introduces many topics surrounding transgender people, including the psychological, physical, and social processes transgender people undergo; the unique experiences of transgender people; and the complexities of gender.

Transgender History, by Susan Stryker. Berkeley, CA: Seal Press, 2008.

An examination of transgender history from the mid-twentieth century to current times.

Transitions of the Heart: Stories of Love, Struggle and Acceptance by Mothers of Transgender and Gender Variant Children, edited by Rachel Pepper. Berkeley, CA: Cleis Press, 2012.

A collection of stories by mothers of trans* children about their experiences with their child's gender transition.

Trans-Kin: A Guide for Family and Friends of Transgender People, edited by Eleanor A. Hubbard and Cameron T. Whitley. Winter Park, FL: Bolder Press, 2012.

An anthology of stories by friends, family, and allies of transgender people about their experiences.

Films

Gendernauts: A Journey Through Shifting Identities, by Monika Traut. New York: First Run Features, 1999.

Follows the lives of a group of trans* people living outside of their prescribed gender identities. Participants include performance artist Annie Sprinkle and Internet activist Sandy Stone.

Transgeneration, by Jeremy Simmons and Thairin Smothers. Sundance Channel, 2005.

Eight-episode documentary series depicting the lives of four transgender college students as they transition.

Gay and Lesbian Alliance Against Defamation (GLAAD)

323-933-2240

www.glaad.org

A leading organization that works with news media, entertainment media, social media, and cultural institutions to shape the public's view of LGBTQ people.

HuffPost Gay Voices

www.huffingtonpost.com/gay-voices

A website that publishes articles from a variety of viewpoints about LGBTQ issues.

Human Rights Campaign

800-777-4723

www.hrc.org

One of the largest LGBTQ advocacy organizations in the United States. The Resources and Issues sections on the website are very useful for understanding the current status of all LGBTQ rights and for finding additional information.

LEGAL RIGHTS

Get Equal

www.getequal.org

An advocacy organization that encourages and helps individuals get involved in their community in order to fight for LGBTQ rights.

Lambda Legal

212-809-8585

www.lambdalegal.org

The oldest and largest national, LGBTQ focused legal organization, Lambda Legal's mission is to achieve full recognition of the civil rights of LGBTQ people and those living with HIV through impact litigation, education, and public policy work.

National Gay and Lesbian Task Force

202-393-5177

www.thetaskforce.org

One of the nation's leading advocacy organizations that works to advance legal rights of the LGBTQ community by training activists, researching and analyzing policy, and keeping the public up to date on legal issues.

U.S. Books

Making Gay History: The Half-Century Fight for Lesbian and Gay Equal Rights, by Eric Marcus. New York: Harper Perennial, 2002.

Incorporating accounts from a large variety of voices—from everyday people to Ellen DeGeneres—this book documents the gay civil rights movement over the past fifty years.

Out in the Country: Youth, Media, and Queer Visibility in Rural America, by Mary L. Gray. New York: NYU Press, 2009.

A look at queer life in rural areas, using the author's personal narratives and expository writing.

Queer America: A People's GLBT History of the United States, by Vicki L. Eaklor. New York: New Press, 2011.

An examination of twentieth century LGBTQ issues and rights, through the lens of LGBTQ people.

Global Perspectives

Love's Rite: Same-Sex Marriage in India and the West, by Ruth Vanita. Basingstoke, U.K.: Palgrave Macmillan, 2005.

Examines the presence of gay marriage in the Hindu foundations of Indian culture and the subtle evolution of opinion regarding homosexuality in India, within the context of the global debate on same-sex marriage.

Tommy Boys, Lesbian Men, and Ancestral Wives: Female Same-Sex Practices in Africa, by Ruth Morgan and Saskia Wieringa. Johannesburg, South Africa: Jacana Media, 2006.

Focuses on the prevalence of homosexual African women, despite the taboo on homosexuality in most African cultures.

Unspeakable Love: Gay and Lesbian Life in the Middle East, by Brian Whitaker. Berkeley: University of California Press, 2006.

A comparative look at the progress and struggles of LGBTQ life in the Arab world to that of LGBTQ life in the Western world.

Films

After Stonewall, directed by John Scagliotti. New York: First Run Features, 1999.

Documentary that looks at the LGBTQ rights movement between the 1969 Stonewall Riots and the turn of the twenty-first century.

Before Stonewall, directed by John Scagliotti. New York: First Run Features, 1986.

Documentary that looks at the LGBTQ rights movement before the Stonewall Riots.

Call Me Kuchu, directed by Malika Zouhali-Worrall and Katherine Fairfax Wright. New York: Cinedigm Entertainment Group, 2012.

Documentary that explores the struggles of the LGBTQ community in Uganda.

Out of the Past: The Struggle for Gay and Lesbian Rights in America, directed and produced by Jeff Dupre, written by Michelle Ferrari. Arlington, VA: PBS, 1998.

Documentary that examines LGBTQ political and social movements in America over the last 400 years.

GLBT National Help Center

National Hotline: 888-843-4564

Youth Hotline: 800-246-7743

www.glnh.org

A hotline and online chat service for LGBTQ people, with a specific line dedicated for youth. Anyone can call, even if they are not in crisis.

National Suicide Prevention Lifeline

800-273-8255

www.suicidepreventionlifeline.org

A telephone and online chat service for those in crisis, as well as other mental health resources.

Substance Abuse and Mental Health Services Administration

U.S. Dept. of Health & Human Services

877-726-4727

www.samhsa.gov

An agency within the U.S. Department of Health that offers a variety of resources and centers with focuses on suicide, bullying, substance abuse, and homelessness, including LGBTQ-specific services.

The Trevor Project

Lifeline: 866-488-7386

www.thetrevorproject.org

A leading national organization in crisis intervention for LGBTQ youth. Services include a suicide hotline, online chat services, text services, and an LGBTQ youth–specific social networking service.

RELIGION

Gay Christian Network

919-786-0000

www.gaychristian.net

Provides a variety of resources, from books to documentaries to a musical, about homosexuality and Christianity. The site also offers online discussion forums and other methods of support.

Websites

Christian Gays

christiangays.com

Articles, chat rooms, and resources on being gay and Christian.

LGBT Faith Tumblr

lgbtfaith.tumblr.com

Writing on the intersection of sexual orientation and faith. Additional resources are also available.

OrthoGays

orthogays.com

Information and resources for gay and lesbian Orthodox Jews.

The Safra Project

safraproject.org

A resource project working on issues related to lesbian, bisexual, and/or transgender women who identify as Muslim religiously and/or culturally.

Books

Homosexuality in Islam: Critical Reflection on Gay, Lesbian, and Transgender Muslims, by Scott Siraj al-Haqq Kugle. Oxford, U.K.: Oneworld Publications, 2010.

Examines the Koran's writings about homosexuality, with an end goal of reconciling homosexuality and Islam.

Unfair: Christians and the LGBT Question, by John Shore. Seattle: CreateSpace Independent Publishing Forum, 2013.

A combination of personal essays by LGBT-identified Christians and essays by Shore about the importance of reconciling homosexuality and Christianity.

What the Bible Really Says about Homosexuality, by Daniel Helminiak. Estancia, NM: Alamo Square Press, 2000.

Biblical scholars analyze the Bible, especially the passages often used to condemn homosexuality, to demonstrate that homosexuality and Christianity are not as at odds as many believe.

Films

For the Bible Tells Me So, by Daniel Karslake. New York: First Run Features, 2007.

Documentary that follows five families of faith as their child comes out and the family must learn to reconcile homosexuality and Christianity. A study guide can be found online.

A Jihad for Love, written and directed by Parvez Sharma. New York: First Run Features, 2008.

Documentary that examines Islam and homosexuality, interviewing people from around the world.

Through My Eyes, directed by Justin Lee. Raleigh, NC: Gay Christian Network, 2009.

Documentary that features young Christians who talk about their struggles in accepting their homosexuality and reconciling with their faith.

Trembling Before G-d, by Sandi Simcha Dubowski. New York: New Yorker Films, 2001.

Documentary that follows lesbian and gay Orthodox Jews who struggle with accepting both their sexuality and their faith.

LGBTQ-Friendly Places of Worship

GLBT Near Me

www.glbtnearme.org

This is a generic LGBTQ-friendly search engine for all types of businesses with a specific filter for places of worship.

Institute for Welcoming Resources

612-821-4397

www.welcomingresources.org

Includes both a search engine for LGBTQ-friendly places of worship and online resources for issues about faith and LGBTQ issues.

Advocates for Youth

202-419-3420

www.advocatesforyouth.org

Their services include online and print resources, policy analysis and advocacy, and outreach initiatives around the country.

Health Initiatives for Youth

415-274-1970

www.hify.org

A multicultural organization whose mission is to improve the health and well-being of underserved young people through youth leadership, popular education, and advocacy, in pursuit of multi-level social change.

Planned Parenthood

Health services: 800-230-7526

Information: 212-541-7800

www.plannedparenthood.org

A leading organization in advocating for and providing sex education and sexual health services.

Websites

Go Ask Alice

goaskalice.columbia.edu

This Columbia University site offers a daily question-and-answer blog about health and sexuality.

Scarleteen

www.scarleteen.com

A plethora of informational articles geared for teens about topics related to healthy sexuality, from anatomy to relationships to sexual politics.

Books

S.E.X.: The All-You-Need-To-Know Progressive Sexuality Guide to Get You Through High School and College, by Heather Corinna. Cambridge, MA: Da Capo Press, 2007.

Covers a wide spectrum of topics about sexuality, from anatomy to STIs to misogyny to deciding to live together. The writing is LGBTQ-inclusive.

Index

Acknowledgments

We wanted to proposition our publisher for fourteen pages in which to properly thank the following individuals, but then gently reminded ourselves that we are not (in this instance) the center of the universe. With that in mind, we would like to extend the biggest thanks possible to the following people, without whom this book would, quite literally, not exist: Dr. Linda Stone Fish, Dr. Justine Shuey, Dr. Sherri Palmer, Alyse Knorr, Tom Montgomery, Erika Lynn, Keanan, Zak, Tyler, Robert, Marianne, PFLAG Charleston, Anna Livia, and all of our magnificent interns. We'd also like to thank Joh, Laurel, Christian, Tonia, LT, Jen, Allison, Kristine, Sandy, Sloan, the entire Faccone family, Steven, Sammy, and Justin Bieber.

To all of the parents and teenagers and twenty-somethings who sat with us and shared their stories and their feedback: you are the reason we are doing this, and simultaneously the reason that we can do this.

To Lisa, for her way with words, her perfectly placed commas, her persistence, and her vision.

And finally, to JL, the hardest-working, most brilliant literary agent on planet Earth: you are our heart and soul.

Kristin's thanks:

To my mom, who worked tirelessly to return to herself, her faith, and her daughter—I love you; to my dad, whose five-foot-seven, 140-pound frame would find the strength to fight the entire world on my behalf; to my sister, who just *gets it*; to my Aunt Theresa, who has never wavered in her ability to speak her mind, to be open to the thoughts of others, and to love fiercely and without hesitation; to Randi, my constant; to Trey, who is always reliably covered in fur; to Jenny, who saves me from both myself and the world each and every day; and to Dannielle, who understands me in ways that no one else can, who works beside me every hour of every day, and who was put on this planet to be my partner in the most ridiculous and profound journey of a lifetime. We can't stop.

Dannielle's thanks:

I'd like to extend the warmest of thank-yous to the people in my life who have inspired me, challenged me, believed in me, and pushed me to work harder than I thought possible. To my friends and family, I cannot thank you enough for all that you do; to Dad, who has made me the person I am so proud to have become and who has taught me everything I know; to Janet, my sister from another mister who is also a cat; to Amanda, Hillary, Zettler, and Brynn who keep me in line, make me LOL, and remind me how to be a good friend; and to Kristin, my accidental life partner and fellow adventurer, who helps me keep my sanity, understands me in ways no one ever will, and who I can't imagine my life without. We won't stop.